SIX MINUTE SEX!

Maintaining Passion and Nurturing Intimacy in Long Term Relationships

Written By: Cindi Seddon

www.sizzlenotfizzle.com

Illustrated by: Ricky Villanueva Castillo
https://www.fiverr.com/rickycastillo

ISBN: 9781738770007

Contents

Next, checkout **SIZZLENOTFIZZLE.com** (launching February 14, 2023) for our weekly podcast, and more fun ideas and ways to contribute to stronger connections between you and your life partner. We will be looking to publish a book every year based on the stories submitted that fit under the title of "The True Story of How We Met!" If you have a story to share about how you met your lifelong partner, look for "How To Submit Our Story" on the website. Sounds like fun!

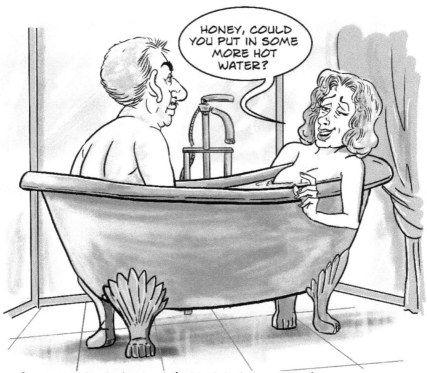

Why You Need To Read the Whole Book - Cover to Cover

Note to all readers! Don't skip through to Chapter 1 - there is a lot of dialogue before that, and everything connects. Be sure to read **The WHOLE THING**, right from the very beginning through to the very end, not in one sitting necessarily, but don't skip even one page!!

Why?

Because I am a storyteller. And in this book I weave our tapestry of tales that revolve around the actual "day to day living" part of living with life long partners. My stories are true (I was there!), and from the many conversations I have had with others, my readers will relate to the diddies I tell. These stories almost always have some kind of fun, silly or ridiculous aspect to them that will make you laugh out loud! However, they also include some of the challenges, roadblocks and sadnesses we have faced together, surviving losses and living through passionless droughts, where the words "in sickness and in health" are really put to the test.

But most of all, there is a good dose of hope woven throughout these pages- hope that love lasts and continues to nurture us, hope that passion lasts throughout the ebb and flow of long term relationships, hope that we, as a couple, will always prevail despite the raucous winds that rock our boats. And all of these intangible elements of our lives together can form a rock hard foundation that not just survives, but thrives!

As I weave this graphic, my goal is to help committed long term relationship partners better understand why, in the long part of the "long term", we must always choose each other, even in times of grief and sorrow, sadness and anger, loss of delight and dark lonely times. As well, by reading this book, it might just re-ignite a passion you share with the person you chose to spend your whole life with that may have cooled down to just a flicker. These stories weave together the journey I have been on for over 40 years.

That is why you should read the whole thing - because it forms a big picture and weaves stories of other long term relationship couples that have also survived and thrived.

You will notice as you read, that the font changes throughout the book. That is done on purpose, as I weave personal stories about Kevin and I (and sometimes our kids and friends) throughout the text. Our personal stories are told in italics, and are designed to compliment the on going text of the book. Sometimes I include lessons I have learned, and sometimes it just makes sense to tell the story. There are funny stories, hard stories, stories of perseverance and stories of tough times we have had in our relationship. The point of writing in this way, for me, is to reinforce that life is a series of stories, some good, others not so good, all woven together into a strong but pliable, warm and welcoming blanket that really gives me great comfort. I hope you enjoy reading as much as I have enjoyed writing.

I just did it again, read the book again that is, for perhaps the 50th time, and it still makes me laugh in some places, and cry in others. As I finish this project (do we ever finish?), my new pup, Lovely (yes that's her name) sits at my feet, sleeping and being cute, following me down the hall every time I take a break, checking to see if I am ready to move around a bit with her, and I am again reminded and inspired by the possibilities that are naturally built into love - good strong steady unpredictable love, playful love, soulful love -the kind of love that rocks your world and gentles your soul. The kind of love that I share with Kevin, my life partner; the kind of love I have for my now grown children; the kind of love I cherish in the relationships with friends and family. I have truly found the magic key to the kingdom - sounds pretty sappy I know, but this journey starts with a dog and ends with a dog.

Starts with the Story of a Dog

We lost our beautiful dog Goldilocks on April 22, 2021. On April 21 she told me it was time for her to go. I listened and then did one of the hardest, most compassionate things I have ever done. I let her go. She fell asleep in my arms as she moved into her final goodnight when her energy changed from this world to whatever comes next. She was so remarkable from the moment we met until the moment we said farewell.

I came across her by way of a happy surprise in 2009, the same way all my dogs have come to me. She was 2 ½ years old and had been a mother 5 times. We saved her from that life, and she in turn gave herself to people completely. She became a certified therapy dog, and I would take her to work (I was a high school principal in an Alternate school) where she would connect with the kids and the staff and make everyone feel better. She had a sense about people that I had never seen in a dog. Often I would be involved in very difficult meetings with young adults who were struggling, and often their parents were there as well. Goldie learned to sense when someone in the meeting was having a hard time, and she would sit outside my office door. My secretary came to know that when Goldie stood outside my closed office door, someone inside needed comforting. My secretary would knock and open the door, and in would come Goldie. She would move directly to the someone in the room who needed comforting (never to me) and she would plunk her head on their lap. I learned to tell many surprised people that this was our school's therapy dog, and she was letting me know that, by putting her head on their lap, she understood that something was troubling them, and that she was there to relieve the burden. There was no need for them to tell anyone in the room what the sadness or concern was. Goldie was just providing love and comfort. I would then tell that person that, in a couple of minutes, she was going to lie down on their feet. Sure enough, this happened every time. The meeting would soften immediately, and in every instance, we would be able to get through some hard topics and plan forward in a positive way. She was able to raise the level of trust in the room, and I was so very grateful to be able to work with her in this way.

However, she never let us forget that she was a dog first, and carried out all sorts of mischief and fun in her long life with us. One day, quite out of character for her, she broke into the new cat food bag and ate 10 pounds out of the 15 pound bag - a sort of self serve buffet! We were not only shocked, but we were pretty upset about her behavior. However, the poor girl was so sick! She had all sorts of intestinal trouble for a couple of days but she never did anything like that again!! I know that we were lucky to have her in our lives.

So, what does this have to do with Six Minute Sex you ask? Well, the deep love and intimacy Kevin and I shared with each other affected our entire living sphere, and Goldie not only felt our mutual devotion, but she came to want to be included in hugs and dances and games and teasings. In retrospect, this was true for all of our dogs! Goldie would get in between us when we were having a moment together, dancing to some favorite tune or just hugging each other. She would dance around when we became playful with each other and she would try to crawl into our skin when one of us was being comforted by the other as we worked through some sadnesses. She really wanted to bring more joy, or at least more peace, to any *situation. That seemed to be her role during her lifetime. I miss her, and it took me a long while to be ready to move forward, but here I am with our new little Lovely, and my heart is full again.*

Thank you for being interested in reading this book. My hope is that you find it engaging all the way through, funny in some places, sad in others, and that it leaves you with a feeling of hope for your future, and reasons for you and your partner to seriously consider spicing up your intimate lives together!

Thanks to?? WELL, EVERYONE!!!

Had the initial idea for this book not been met with such laughter and interest, I would likely never have pursued it. Had people not been patient, yet still asking about the project for over a decade, and then open to reading it, I likely never would have pursued it. Had my husband Kevin not endorsed my efforts each time I went back to it, again I likely would neve have pursued it. Had my youngest daughter not finally been old enough to be too shocked, embarrassed or perhaps even turned off by the idea of Six Minute Sex (by her parents) to offer her expertise on the social media front for pushing this book out, again, unlikely that I would have carried on...But here we are! The support, the curiosity and the interest was like an elixir for me. Every little smile, every giggle, every question about this book's progress told me I was on to something. The fact that, when I read the original draft script, 10 plus years after I wrote it and it still made me laugh in places, prompted that little voice in me to say "GO FOR IT!" So THANK YOU, circle of friends, family and influencers, for being my best encouragers, and for believing that I had a story to tell. It's been a complete blast, with definitely more in store!

My Long Journey: The Writing of Six Minute Sex

Writing this book has been a project undertaken over many years, and now when people ask, "Oh, you're writing a book?", I answer, "Yes, for the 6th or 7th time now - just hoping I can get it right this time and finish!". So here it is - in its final form!

I think I wrote the first draft in 2009. Initially, I expected a publisher to pick it up after I had completed most of the first draft because it was such a great idea, with a lot of fun thrown in. I diligently sent it, by snail mail, to many publishing houses. Snail Mail - that's all I knew how to use, and back then most publishers would only accept draft documents on paper. However, after numerous rejections I decided to put it aside, even though I had told many friends about it, and they said they were just waiting for the book to come out in print. My cheering section!

Time went by, we grew older, parents died, kids grew up, friends came down with various physical and mental health ailments, some died, most survived, and still I did not go back to this project. Through it all, Kevin and I stayed in love and to be fair, did a pretty good job at the six minute thing most of the time. While there were still times of drought, famine and being too tired, we never lost our passion for each other. Then one day in 2018, for the first time in 10 years, I was called back for a second mammogram.

And yes, I had the dreaded disease. F***

The second toughest thing about all of this journey was the waiting - knowing what the outcome was going to be, but having to wait for confirmation. I wanted to scream it out to the world and the heavens, "I have breast cancer" I wanted to grab it, physically, and squeeze the life out of it. But I had to wait and wait for confirmation of the suspected results.

However the toughest, REALLY the toughest part of this whole thing was having to tell our kids that I had breast cancer. They knew that their grandmother (my mother) and aunty (my sister) had it, they knew about it, they knew I went for a mammogram every year for a health check, but having cancer myself felt like I was setting my own kids up for the same hideous disease, because I have girls. But a funny (in the weird way of funny, not haha funny) thing happened when we told them. Sure, there were a few tears, but mostly there was curiosity. Of course I was going the traditional route, of course it was chemo, radiation reconstruction etc, and no I wasn't feeling sick just tired, and I wasn't really scared, just mad, furious in fact. But then we realized this - our children had never known anyone who died of breast cancer! Not one fatality from this form of the disease itself. My mother died of all sorts of ailments, and my sister is a 20 year plus breast cancer survivor. My kids had no concern that I might die. Thank God for children!

And then I realized how far we have come in our fight against this hideous disease - and although the cancer was diagnosed as aggressive and invasive, I knew I was going to survive it. So, I went through the full regimen, bilateral mastectomy with immediate reconstruction (that's both breasts removed and implants put in), sixteen weeks of chemo, or poison being poured into my body to fight the stronger poison that was already in it. Trouble during the healing process with the wound on the left side refusing to heal caused delays in both chemo and radiation. The chemo finally started after the implant on the cancer side had been taken out, healed, and a skin stretcher, like a placeholder, was put in. Then when that did not heal, it too was taken out and I had to heal again. So, I was quite deformed and I put on quite a bit of weight. I walked in the forest every day, usually alone with my beloved dog Goldie. I had to take a long leave from work. I tried to learn Italian to avoid chemo brain but I couldn't retain the new learning. My dad died. My oldest flunked out of 2nd year engineering because she felt so overwhelmed watching me go through this (once they heard her story they let her back in. She is now a mechanical engineer). Eight surgeries later I just hated giving updates to my circle of family and friends because, let's face it, at some point people don't want to read about any more bad news! I was grateful for the scores of people that did kind and lovely things for me and my family. The food, the incredible and delicious food that showed up, that I didn't have to think about, all ready and beautifully prepared for me and my family represented acts of love from friends and coworkers. Flowers that brightened my days and weeks, gift certificates, special and loving hand written messages and cards, taking time to walk with me in the forest, all of these were elixirs for my path to wellness. It was abundance, and it went on for a very long time. As well, I was so grateful for my husband and my kids. I was grateful, everyday, to wake up on this side of the grass!!

But guess what! We still found a way to express our physical love for each other. And yes, we could still both be super relaxed in six minutes. I guess that's what all that therapy in our 30's readied us *for - healing from cancer. I wish I could tell you that it was hard for six months, but in fact it was close to 5 times as long before things really sorted themselves out. I went through having boobs that betrayed me (my own breasts that grew cancer), to having Foobs (fake breasts, implants that refused to let my skin heal), to single breasted and scared (deformed and not beautiful), and now I have MOBO'S (My Own Boobs) or BFB's (belly fat boobs); breasts made up of my own belly fat through the absolute wonders of modern surgery - and almost every woman's dream! The incredibly gifted surgeons took the fat from my belly/abdomen, flipped it up somehow and built breasts - incredible! It was certainly no picnic getting here, and I don't recommend the 8.5 hour surgery that it comes with as well as the 6-8 week recovery, and true to form it took me 8 long weeks, but here I am today. However, I had to wait a long time for the final surgery because, along the way to healing, I got the blood clots (up to 20% of breast cancer patients can get blood clots from the chemo) called pulmonary emboli, but it took quite a while to diagnose, so I got very sick. Clots were in one artery in my lungs, pneumonia was in the other, so I was out for another long recovery from pulmonary emboli while still waiting for the big MOBO surgery. As well, I became concerned that I had trouble retaining information. I knew that chemo brain was a real thing, however word retrieval was problematic from time to time, so more specialists did some investigation and the results showed that I had suffered from T.I.A's (OMG REALLY???) or mini strokes. While they were unable to time date when they had occurred, it was clear that I had suffered multiple mini strokes! All I could think was "what next?"*

Towards the end of this journey, I did finally and a little sadly retire from a career that was so wonderful, so rewarding and a gift from the universe - I retired from education. I was a teacher and administrator for over 30 years, and I am so very grateful to every person I was lucky to cross paths with: students, parents, grandparents, colleagues, professional friends, and everyone in between! What an incredible ride!

Today's health update: at the time of writing this, I am 4 + years cancer free, and I need to get to 5 years cancer free for the best survival rates. I run, I bike, I paddle and I ski - those are my chosen favorites. I run alone, I bike, paddle and ski regularly, season permitting, with Kevin, and sometimes with the girls. Kevin and I are both learning to paddleboard, and I still walk regularly in the forest. I have shed the extra pounds that chemo and COVID helped me put on. I camp a bit and I hike a bit. I feel happy - but to be fair, I have always been a pretty happy person. I have learned I need to reach out more to the people I care about because communication and friendship is a 2 way street. I'm not sure why I haven't picked up with my Italian Language instruction that I started on. Perhaps one day soon I will just start again!

But when I think back over this journey, I think that things were easier for me BECAUSE of Six Minute Sex, because we kept working at it, because I was able to get all of the goodness that comes with regular intimacy. I like to think I got off lucky from the deadly disease of cancer, and I think it's because I really try to live with some pretty good health habits every day, and remind myself to enjoy!

The Story of How it All Started

So, whadaya mean, Six Minute Sex?
What's that?
Why do ya wanna talk about that in a book?
Well, not "what's that " but rather "why", or even "why bother"?
Good Questions! Well, here's the story.

It really all started in 2009. My life partner, Kevin, was with me at our best and favorite adult summer retreat (no children under 14 allowed, and no pets!!), Yellow Point Lodge, located on Vancouver Island in British Columbia, where we had been going for many years, always at the same time of year. This unique and magical place, owned by Richard and Sandy Hill, is the birthplace of many adventurous ideas I have come to know, and it really is the start of this story of a book called Six Minute Sex!

As it happened, we met and became fantastic friends with a sizable group of people who had also been going to Yellow Point Lodge, at the same time of year as us. We used to sit around the fire near the ocean in the evening visiting, singing, telling jokes and tall tales, and one night after maybe a little bit of wine after dinner , the subject turned to sex...well, not exactly the act of sex, but rather the frequency of sex in our long term realtionships. Gales of laughter could be heard coming from the fire as we teased each other and joked about the frequency of lovemaking in our long term relationships. At one point, thinking to make a joke and issue a bit of a challenge, I said, "Well, Kevin and I can do it in 6 minutes!" Whoops of laughter rang out, challenges and "ho-ho-ho's" and from then on, the idea of six Minute

*Sex took on a life of its own! This actually led us to wonder if in fact we **could** start and finish, all in, in 6 minutes, so, like any fun seeking couple, we started timing ourselves and guess what we found out? It could be done! All in!!*

On the heels of that, we started brainstorming everything that might fit into a theme in a book called "Six Minute Sex! So, for a while we just played with the idea of anything 6. This is what we came up with:

1. The Book itself - Six Minute Sex
2. Six chapters
3. Six pages per chapter
4. Six days a week!
5. The six greatest love songs, or the six greatest songs to make love to
6. The six best date night ideas
7. Safe Six - for during COVID times
8. And for newly "In Lover" ers - EVERY Six minutes! Whoot whoot

Some of these ideas, as you may notice, have stuck, some have become pages on our website SIZZLENOTFIZZLE.COM (launching February 14, 2023 have a look), while others are just so ridiculous they have been abandoned! But we had fun brainstorming and then playing out their feasibility.

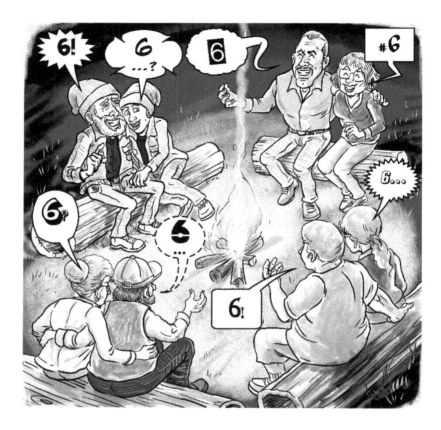

Who knew?

Whether this idea caught on because of its alliteration, or because it was a funny idea, the whole idea of Six Minute Sex became a topic of some interest with our summer friends, and then over time, with our winter friends and other friends. Before long, I started *just talking* about writing a book about Six Minute Sex, and very shortly after that, a friend said to me, "Well if you don't write it, I will!!" Thus the book Six Minute Sex was launched, and the writing began! Thank you Yellow

Point Lodge and my good, good friends!! Again, that was back in 2009!

What I found out, whenever I brought this topic up with other adults, is that there was an awful lot of interest in the idea itself. And as I talked about the notion of Six Minute Sex, I began to more clearly define my interest in this topic. Like others, I was not interested in racing to a "sex deadline" to prove it could be done. Instead, as conversations became more personal, I learned that for many of us lifers who were deeply connected with one partner for many years, me included, sex was not really all that frequent. And it wasn't that we were no longer interested in each other, we just weren't that interested in the investment of making time and taking the energy for sex and intimacy. Why, you ask? Here are some of the reasons I heard:

1. Access - that warm body is always there! We could engage intimately anytime (or maybe later?)!
2. Busy with something or nothing, or just distracted
3. Achy sore body and bones
4. Having something that needs to be done soon
5. Kids/relatives/babies/parents/friends around
6. Different "time to get up" or "time to go to bed" times

So I started to ask questions about that, and to do a little research, and I figured out that it wasn't that we didn't want to have sex, we just didn't want uncomfortable sex, or the long hot sex of our early realtionship, when things might just go on for a very long time, and the idea of short sex was not that enticing, mostly because it wasn't satisfying. And if we thought that all sex had to be like the sex of our early, younger realtionship, we weren't really interested. Those 45-60 minute sessions (or longer?) just did not hold the same interest for us in our more senior years. Then I began to read about all of the health benefits (yes -LOTS!) from regular sex and intimate moments, which actually becomes more important as time goes by and as we age. And the idea of Six Minute Sex actually started making a lot of sense. The longer we know one another the shorter our sessions in the sack become, but often they don't seem to be as satisfying. And so the frequency decreases. So I wondered, what would it take to kindle an interest that met the following criteria:

1. Short, as in not too long - you decide
2. Mutually satisfying - not a chore
3. Includes a high level of comfort
4. Guaranteed distraction free
5. Includes a notable element of fun, freedom, and whimsy, and finally
6. Includes a desire for both parties to invest in our future good health for ourselves and each other. That, as well as a promise that rushing along would be okay! And we would BOTH benefit!

Sex, after a long long time, can feel a bit like a chore or an activity in which we are expected to engage. And for some, an element of boredom sometimes creeps in, or achy bones and muscles begin to interfere with the pleasure - a whole host of issues can arise. Bodies change shape and consistency, and for some it becomes less comfortable being naked in front of even a mirror, let alone our life partner. But we can change the parameters to better fit our lives! We are ALLOWED to change the rules and parameters anytime. After all, it's just between us!

This book is finally here because...

While I am so curious about relationships, specifically loving, romantic relationships; relationships that last a lifetime where the partners commit to a long term intimate bond, I am captured by the idea of Six Minute Sex with a long term partner even after a really long time, and I am even more fascinated when the relationship survives for years and years, and the loving romantic connection never dies. Aren't you? How does that happen? Because almost all relationships begin with two strangers meeting one another. And although they start as complete strangers, they end up over a long time willing to die for one another, their love for each is so deep and true. How does this happen? Magic I say!!!

Being a half of one of those couples, I am at the same time curious about the ebb and flow of intimacy, and how we feel about one another, and how, after years together, the impact of daily life can so easily erode the passion and the nurturing of intimacy - and I am shocked that we can so easily lose each other to mediocrity. In this book, I fight against complacency and the dulling of the senses and passions that once burned so brightly and consistently. I fight against being lulled into a sober, comfortable kind of love, the kind that feels like putting on an old and comfortable pairs of shoes, or a warm comfy sweater on a chilly day, and losing the intoxicating feelings and emotions that come with passionate love - putting off for tomorrow what we did not do today, but should have! But putting it off because that resource, that passionate, that loving warm body will be there tomorrow, and tomorrow after that. However, I have learned that for most of us who boast to others about the number of years we have been together, we have moved from a wild teeter-totter, roller coaster of love and sex and emotion and passion and romance to a softer landing, a quietness together that, while comforting, needs some razzle dazzle shaking up too. We need a reminder from each other how much we matter, and what's worth fighting for. Relationship, intimacy, passion, sexual fun and pleasure, friendship, connectedness - that's what we fight for - that's what we want to keep. And I encourage you to fight for that too!

So, when you think about the odds of having met your true love, do you wonder, "How did we even get together? Fate? Providence? Or just good luck? How does it happen? Strangers meet. In a zillion different manners. And sometimes there is a spark, which can ignite into a hot flame. And sometimes that hot flame cools a bit and settles into commitment and relationship, and then, settles even further into a committed couple who start a new life together, and then sometimes that committed couple consummate their commitment and seal their future legacy with children of their own making. It is a remarkable thing, this journey of 2 strangers becoming one unit, and then a family. But just as complex as relationships are amongst humans, we are not the only species that mate for more than just procreation. In the animal kingdom, 3-5% mate for life! For example, the gray wolf, the bald eagle, prairie voles and swans (to name just a few) mate for life. In these relationships, the male helps with raising the young. Some of these lifetime couples dance together throughout their lives, some sing to one another, while others work as a team to keep their little ones safe.

Other species, like the gibbon, choose a partner they mostly stick with, but Chase tail-less monkeys cheat on one another, and sometimes separate for good.

> Staying faithful can be a struggle for most animals. For one, males are hardwired to spread their genes and females try to seek the best dad for their young. Also, monogamy is costly because it requires an individual to place their entire reproductive investment on the fitness of their mate. Putting all their eggs in one basket means there's a lot of pressure on each animal to pick the perfect mate, which, as humans know, can be tricky. (livescience.com)

There are many similarities in love and lust between human beings and the rest of the animal kingdom - we all crave some form of companionship.

One of the most interesting and enjoyable things I like to do is asking people how they met. I think I could write a book on that alone: maybe I will! I just love those stories!! The newly formed couple have been raised separately by different adults in parental roles, in traditional or non-traditional settings, usually, teaching and practicing 2 different sets of values and ways of living. They may even have been raised far apart from one another and definitely have different memories and experiences. They meet, something sparks, and they begin to fall into passionate love, where the two of them want to know everything about the other, they want to spend time together, they want to be intimate with one another, and then some decide to make a lifetime commitment to each other. While research suggests that the divorce rate has sometimes exceeded 50% over the last 40 years (depending on many variables such as first, second or third time married, income, education to name a few "yourdivorcequestion.org 2021"), those that stay together acknowledge that they **want** to be together, they **want** an identity as a couple and in the end feel safer and are willing to give more to their partner (Dr. Scott Stanley, 2021).

Remember - Anything can get in the way of your happiness and the intimate connection you have with your partner - Anything. But it's a two sided coin. Nothing can get in the way of your happiness and the intimate connection with your partner - Nothing. It's all in how you let life affect you.

When I met Kevin I was 22 years old.

It was a beautiful summer evening in June, 1982, and I was at my brother Scott and sister in law Lorraine's home having been invited for dinner. We were sitting outside, enjoying the feeling of being full and basking in each other's company when Scott said that we had been invited to a wedding reception, essentially a party, with some of his friends that I knew as well. We soon decided to attend the soiree, so off we went to a wedding reception where I was sure to know many of the guests, but had no idea who the bride and groom were.

Shortly after arriving, I spotted an interesting looking guy sitting kind of on his own and I whispered to my sister in law - "Hey! See that guy sitting over there? The blond guy with the beard? He's kinda cute and I want to go meet him, but I don't want it to look like I am picking him up, so come with me." Being a good sport, Lorraine came with me so I could meet the man who shortly became the love of my life, and much later became my life partner, the father of our children and (probably was always) the best guy in the world! That night was magical - the wedding reception was fun because we went from the reception to a house party not too far away, and continued the celebration. My new found love interest, Kevin (but I kept calling him Keith - couldn't keep his name straight) had a motorcycle upon which we rode across town, me in a halter dress and high heels, and he in his denim and corduroy outfit. When the party finally got shut down around dawn, we hopped back on his motorcycle and rode back to my place. On the way my helmet fell off (it just came undone and popped off!) and Kevin had to circle his way back to pick it up and affix it more tightly around my chin. Once we got to my place we drank some delicious sparkling mineral water and promptly fell asleep in each other's arms on the couch!

When I was awoken at 11:00 am by my brother Scott wanting to pick me up so I could get my car, I realized that my halter dress was somewhat disheveled!! Whoops!!! I straightened it up, said yes to the ride to my car, explained to Kevin what I was going to do, invited him to stay and help himself to coffee or whatever, and left, saying I would return soon if he wanted to stick around. I remember saying to Scott and Lorraine that there was a really cute guy on my couch and that I hoped he would stay until I returned. Well, guess what!! He did! I remembered that it was Father's Day that Sunday and knew at some point I would venture to my parents' home for dinner, but Kevin and I spent the day together on the balcony of my little apartment, looking out at other apartments that lined the block, and talked and talked and talked, and when he left me, he had my phone number in his pocket and a promise to call. That was how we met.

In our conversation I knew that he had planned a 2 week motorcycle trip to Mexico, leaving in about 10 days. I was a full time university student close to the start of my education journey, and in the middle of my summer semester. We saw each other a few times prior to him leaving on his adventure, and the night before he left we had both shyly and cautiously used the "L" word when we talked about how we thought this thing we were in was going.

Ten days and lots of phone calls later Kevin arrived back having finished his excellent adventure, and the romance was ON!!! We were in it to win it! I spent the rest of that semester attending all my lectures and classes, taking notes, not remembering a thing, reliving my times with Kevin, just waiting to see him again. What a waste of money that semester was for me. I don't think I learned anything, but somehow I passed my courses!! I had completely and totally fallen into romantic, hot sexy love.

So when we started out, I was a student at university studying to be a teacher, he was a tradesman. I drove a VW beetle, he drove a Landcruiser. He lived in a nice house with a roommate and I lived in an apartment. I weighed about 145 pounds. I thought I was fat. He thought I was wonderful! He knew music, he had a tape deck in his truck, he rode a motorcycle, he was cute and funny and kind. He was generous and made me feel special. And he was fun to be with. I thought he must be blind! When we got married 11 years later, I was a teacher with a sensible car, we owned a home and lived in the tiny suite downstairs, renting out the top 2 floors to pay the mortgage. On my wedding day I topped the scale at 276 pounds. Well, I thought, if that's not a reason to back out of this commitment, what is? There was no backing out. Not for Kevin. Not for me either! Thirty years after the wedding we have survived birthing and raising 2 beautiful children (our greatest accomplishment!), career changes, parents dying, breast cancer, surgeries, renovations, owning sailboats and RV's, moving, unimaginable sadnesses, but we still have each other, Thank God. And to be truthful, I think that the playing out of the idea of Six Minute Sex and nurturing the intimacy, has helped our relationship in untold ways!

So, welcome to
SIX MINUTE SEX!
MAINTAINING PASSION AND NURTURING INTIMACY IN LONG TERM RELATIONSHIPS

I hope you enjoy the read, and change up your ride a bit! I hope you get to laugh out loud in some places, and I hope that the book leaves you with more than you started with! While there is a lot to laugh about, each chapter has its serious component - the parts that talk about feeling shame or embarrassment, the frustration we sometimes feel towards the one we are supposed to love most, the challenge for all of us when life gets in the way. My research has taken me along a few different paths discussing how we all can nurture the intimacy between each other and build on what works best for the both of us. While I use many personal stories, as well as examples I have been given permission to share, I treat these stories tenderly and with the great respect and the passion they deserve. Remember- nothing is as funny, as unreal, or as shocking as real life experiences.

And here's just some really good advice!

Pay Attention To These 13 Win Win Strategies for Long Term Relationship Success

Dr John Gottman (2017) says:

Fact: Couples who…

1. Say "I love you" every day and mean it
2. Kiss one another passionately for no reason
3. Give surprise romantic gifts
4. Know what turns their partners on and off erotically
5. Are physically affectionate, even in public

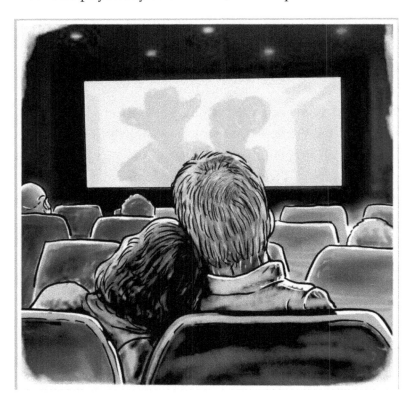

6. Keep playing and having fun together
7. Cuddle
8. Make sex a priority, not the last item of a long to-do list
9. Stay good friends
10. Can talk comfortably about their sex life
11. Have weekly dates
12. Take romantic vacations
13. Are mindful about turning toward each other

…have an amazing sex life, based on this and other studies of over 3000 couples over 4 decades.

Additionally, couples who do not have a great sex life everywhere on the planet are not doing these things. (2017 - Building a Great Sex Life is not Rocket Science)

When I take my score and Kevin's score out of 13, we each hit about a 6! And not the same 6 either! I don't even know how that could happen, but anyway!

So, even if you find your score seems low, the fact that you hit the scoreboard at all counts! Feel comforted that you are a part of a group that is interested in maintaining passion and nurturing intimacy in your long term relationship with your best person!

Chapter 1

SO MANY REASONS WHY SIX MINUTE SEX IS GREAT - TAKE ADVANTAGE OF THE HEALTH BENEFITS!

There's an old saying that my friend used to say every once in a while, and it still makes me smile.

Marriage is like a hot bath. After a while, it just ain't that hot anymore.

And it doesn't matter how much hot water you add to try to warm it up, it just is NEVER gonna be that hot ever again.

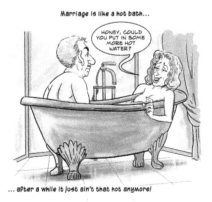

Marriage is like a hot bath...

HONEY, COULD YOU PUT IN SOME MORE HOT WATER?

... after a while it just ain't that hot anymore!

Intimacy and passion and long term primary relationship - who could have predicted that, for some of us, this would be our biggest challenge of aging together.

My husband, Kevin and I have been together in a monogamous relationship for over 40 years; but did not marry until the 11th year. We've had children come and stay, pets come and go. We have taken care of aging and ailing parents and at some point in the future, we will likely welcome grandchildren into our family. Until fairly recently, we both still worked full time and we've always believed that there might be a time when we make enough money to have some left over at the end of the month, although we are not there yet. It has been a while since we have stood on soccer fields in the rain or waited at the sides of the swimming pools and dance classes for the lessons to end, but other consuming hobbies and events quickly took their place. However, we are not yet empty nesters - completely.

We are no longer the hope of change for the future, rather we hope that our children are. We are now the supporters. When I first started this project, we may still have been able to have a baby, but that chapter is long over. We are in the same position that hundreds of thousands of couples are in all around the world; we are not old, but we know that some behaviors are timed out forever (such as me wearing a bikini!) We are not a young couple, but we still notice when the other partner looks particularly good.

Kevin can still make me laugh until I cry, spontaneously, and he also makes me crazy enough to consider committing murder. We move together like a tapestry in motion where independent parts rely on the gestalt of the complete picture to have it all make sense. Rhythm and rhyme. He is mine and I am his, and in this singularity we are committed to each other, choosing a monogamous partnership in our intimacy. We love each other forever and for always, and we are in love with each other most of the time. After over 4 decades, we are pretty happy with that.

Thinking back to the beginning years, like most new couples, we spent the first 18 months full of physical curiosity for each other with no satiation in sight. I remember going through an entire summer semester in University with almost no clue what was going on in my classes, but waiting out every minute until I could see him again. I remember, so vividly, not the moments but the intensity – the intensity of committing and falling in love, of negotiating two lives and life plans into one household, of planning and believing that this was all just too good. I remember wondering if it was even possible for someone to love this deeply. The first 18 months, I think, should always be just like magic.

But 18 months pales as we age together. And the more I talk about this to other couples in the same situations, the clearer it is that a pattern of less regular physical intimacy as we age together seems to be more common than not. That hot bath just never gets that hot again. Adding hot water helps for sure, however for many of us, we have to remember to add that heat, warm things up artificially if necessary, but keep adding heat!! There are peaks and valleys, for sure in terms of sharing intimacy and passion with each other, and dare I say, deserts of loneliness. But that level of intimacy, that level of sharing, of taking the plunge, of losing yourself in one another, even briefly, is so very necessary for managing life.

Depending on which national or international norm you want to believe, the range of intimate relations between long term couples spans between 2-3 times per month to 2-3 times per week. When we read something like that, many of us feel inadequate and wonder how on earth any long term couple can manage, or even want to manage intimacy 2-3 times per week. WOW. REALLY? "How do they do that?" we wonder. "Why do they still do that?" However, some studies have found that once or twice a month is closer to the average. What, then, is getting in the way for those of us that fall short of the norms?? This is where I think we might err: the last time we couldn't get enough of each other was young people's sex. Young love sex. The sex was frequent, curious, engaging and long. Most of us don't want that kind of sex anymore. We want what I call "old people's sex"! Time for a transision to sex that feels invigorating! Old people's sex! Fast, Fun, Fulfilling and Frequent. That sounds WAY more appealing than the sex of our youth in long term relationships.

Most common complaints about what gets in the way of our "couples" time together include:

Kids

Schedules

Too tired

Headache, back ache, other aches and pains (yes, still used regularly)

Not enough energy

Gotta get up too early

Dog, cat (or other pet)

Just don't feel like it

Good (crummy) program on the TV

Phone, computer, messaging, texting, etc.

Takes too long

And then perhaps, just perhaps, these:

Loss of excitement

Embarrassment of body changes (put on weight, take off weight, illness, disability, etc)

Shyness

Awkwardness (not being as bendable and flexible)

It won't be good for me

The kids might hear - used many times in the RV and the boat, and even when we realized that we shared a non soundproof wall with one of the children's bedrooms - time for the cork noise deadener on each side of the wall (it looks great painted).

And yes, I call them complaints rather than excuses. I think that many couples are interested in the IDEA of intimacy with their partner. Why wouldn't we be? We sleep better, our skin is clearer, we have less stress and in fact are able to better handle the stress we do have in our lives, we burn calories, we relax. In fact, some health experts suggest that our beds are a great piece of exercise equipment for mild to moderate activity. According to a multitude of the articles that have been published over the last several years relating to the health benefits of regular sex, we have to ask, "why is it that we have to be talked into such an enjoyable activity?"

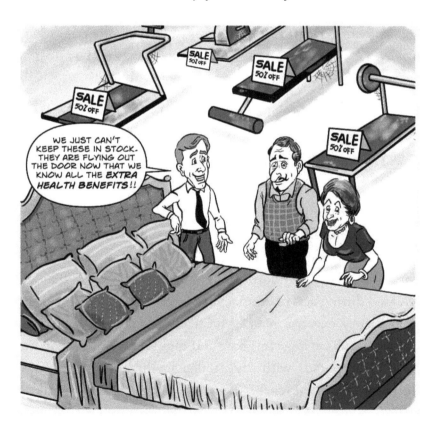

Stop thinking this is a race to the finish line and learn what you can do to keep you and your partner healthy! Never mind the 10,000 steps. Your heart will thank you for your renewed interest in intimate adventures. Also, as we age, our bodies change and for some, they feel some shyness or even shame and/or embarrassment about how their body has aged. Getting past the spoils of gravity is a challenge, but remember who you are with!!! This is the person committed to you, and you to them, so start slowly and reassure each other along the way! Likely they too show some signs of aging, but does it bother you?? No. You may not have even noticed!

Think of all of the great things we can do for our bodies if we even entertain the idea of a six minute segue before we get up, after work, before dinner (while the pasta is cooking!), or any other time. **EVERYONE has six minutes**…

Based on a number of medical studies around the health benefits of intimacy (Medically reviewed by Timothy J. Legg, Ph.D., CRNP —Updated August 3, 2017), the levels of the hormone oxytocin, endorphins and immunoglobulins that are released during acts of intimacy are better for us than any short term diet or exercise plan. MaClean's Magazine (2009) cites Canadians as the most intimate and regular lovemakers on the planet compared with the Italians, the Americans, the Germans, and the French! Think about that. Perhaps a little healthy competition between countries might well go a long way to building a stronger social structure, and a stronger elder community for our youngsters to use as a model for themselves. According to Dr Parthat Nandi (Healthline 2017), the following is a list of proven benefits from having regular up close and personal contact.

Weight loss
Increased fitness
Improved cardiovascular strength
Boost to immune system
Increased life expectancy
Reduced tensions
Relaxed muscles
Feelings of happiness, contentedness and wellbeing

How can all that be bad for us? But let's be a little practical. OK, so maybe you won't shed pounds quickly, but sex burns calories, and regular sex burns calories regularly and increases cardio strength. And if you think about it, that just makes sense. Heart rate goes up, breathing becomes more rapid, calories are burned. Don't bother trying to figure out how long or how many times you need to engage in order to lose X number of pounds. That's not the point. The part about knowing that you are doing something good for yourself is enough.

For those committed athletes who rise and run early in the morning, think about this. What if you varied your routine, just slightly once or twice a week, and did a little "under cover" time first thing in the morning. What a terrific way to start the day! Worried about not getting enough cardio? Find a steep hill to walk up in the evening. Take your partner, and the dog. Those love hormones released in the morning will last for hours, and your conversations will bring you closer together as a couple. I just said to a girlfriend of mine the other day, after a strenuous hike up a mountain in the early morning - "This is my second favorite way to start the day!" she looked at me, laughed and said "Ya!"

Better and deeper sleep patterns

This magic little hormone is responsible for many great things that occur when falling in love. The love hormone, oxytocin is released in vast quantities during sex, and there seem to be multiple benefits from this little darling. One of them is sleeping better. This is particularly true if orgasm is reached. Again, if you think about it, it makes sense. How many women have looked jealous of their partner when, after an intimate act, their partner seems to have no difficulty catching 40 winks!!!! All muscles relax more deeply. Even 20 minute power naps have the ability to rejuvenate and revive energy levels. In fact, the benefits of oxytocin are remarkable!

The science behind it?

Also called the "love hormone," oxytocin is a naturally occurring hormone and a neurotransmitter that is produced in the hypothalamus and transmitted into the bloodstream by the pituitary gland. The hormone is released during childbirth, sex, and lactation to help reproductive functions. The hormone appears to be present in men, as well. It plays a role in sperm movement and the production of testosterone (Makati Medical

Center,6 Effects of the "Love Hormone" Oxytocin February 7, 2020)

Keep reading!

Increased feelings of intimacy, trust, protection and connection with your partner

Oxytocin is magic! Or rather, if you believe in the magic of love, romance, feelings of closeness and the need to connect, then "O" is magic! The love hormone is known for many startling behaviors that are good for us. And the way to get more of a good thing is to make love more often. Physical love doesn't always have to include intercourse. A friend of mine challenged a group of us to just kiss intimately for six minutes. Six minutes of intimate kissing only. What a challenge. Who knew it was so good for our health?? Even our dental health!!! Deep intimate kissing is excellent foreplay, and I have not yet been able to find one couple who were able to do nothing except kiss for six minutes without things moving forward. No one seems to be able to turn off the heat after igniting the romantic flame which moves things along. Everyone should at least try it!

Once released, oxytocin is held accountable for deeper feelings of love, intimate looseness, protection, trust and feeling safe. Conversations are deeper, trust is strengthened, and we come to rely on each other just a little more. Hugging, kissing, hand holding; the human touch specifically intended for affection can stimulate the production of this hormone. So, what are we waiting for I wonder. Whenever Kevin is spontaneously physically affectionate towards me, I can almost feel the release of oxytocin. I feel special, better looking, more inclined to be affectionate back, and flattered. It just feels good!

Healthier heart

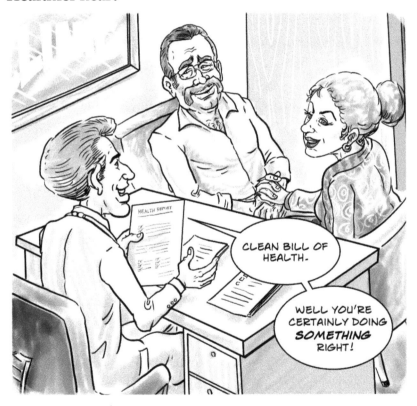

Studies show that regular, REALLY regular intimacy for men reduces their chances of heart attack by up to 50%. That's worth considering.

Reduced risk of Breast Cancer in Women and Prostate Cancer in Men

Not really a surprise, is it? Yes, I know I got it anyway, but perhaps it may have been much more serious? The health benefits of regular intimacy are significant. Like anything that improves with time, couples may not suddenly feel a surge of good health immediately upon increasing their connection times. However, like anything worth pursuing, over time couples and individuals just feel better, look better and find themselves less anxious, less tired, and less stressed, while noticing feelings of increased energy, feelings of well being and satisfaction. What is so very interesting to me is that so many of us are willing to try a new diet to lose weight, begin a new exercise regime to look and feel better, or to try some kind of new vitamin to increase our energy levels, ALL OF WHICH COST MONEY! But like anything out there, we are told by the experts that we must sustain the change. Diets must transform into lifestyles, and exercise routines and vitamin regimens must do the same. All of these changes will infuse good health over time. I urge couples not to overlook the health benefits that their partner can bring them, and that might just be the very best "home remedy" of all.

Pain relief

Yes, those six minutes hold a faster and healthier way to getting rid of those headaches and back pains. As the oxytocin levels increase, so do their endorphins. These endorphins are similar to a runner's high, and pain levels then naturally decrease! No more headache! Imagine that the six minute option is a cure!!

For Women, Strengthening of the Pelvic Floor Muscles

Put simply, no more pee pee leaks when running, laughing or sneezing with regular six minute session routines. No more Kegels Ball exercises. Six minute sessions naturally tighten up those loose and lazy muscles!

While there are a host of other benefits, the point has been made. And really, if you think about it, those health experts are right! Buy a new bed. And some new bedding. Transform your bedroom into the Passion Palace. Call it that! Make a date to tidy the Passion Palace. Lock the dog out. Don't tell the children where you are. They won't miss you for six minutes. Forget the new diet, the juicer you need to buy, the $100 runners and the $100 outfit to go with them. Buy a bed instead. And great pillows! They will last longer, and serve a multitude of needs! Pillows are about the best investment payoff in personal comfort. Pillows are needed every night, 365 days per year. Good pillows will cost only pennies a day and will provide hours of rest and relief. Think of how much you might be currently spending at your favorite coffee shop every week.

Multiply that by 52. Believe me when I tell you that you can get **THE BEST PILLOW IN THE WORLD** for just a fraction of that cost, and enjoy it for hours every night. Think about it.

The diet industry has been making billions of dollars off of us when the answer to our prayers is quite simply where we say our prayers. And the beauty of this is, six minutes is enough. Intimacy does not really need a specific timeframe. There are no "intimacy police" who have stopwatches or rule books. A friend recently told me, "Cindy - we're seniors. Six minutes isn't enough time. We need 7 minutes. Change the title of your book!!" No one is checking to be sure all items on the list are marked off. Sometimes, when we think we need to keep up the energy required for intimacy for 30-40 minutes, or whatever you and your partner remember as a reasonable or required amount of time to have completed the act, neither party can even think about expending that much energy. Or time. It makes us feel tired, too tired to even try. The idea of even starting anything can suck all the air out of the room, but why is that? The truth is that intimacy builds relationships, and the deeper the relationship, the stronger the bond. Strong bonds can endure, in such a healthier way, the challenges that are placed before all of us, the ones that we have no way of predicting, and we need to just live through. As all of us know by now, there are no free rides in life. No one gets off without significant challenges. Throw the timelines and preconceived notions away and enjoy yourselves.

Well, you might ask, "what happens when six minutes is simply not enough??" Great!! Fabulous!! Read chapter 4!! Lots of great information in Chapter 4 for those who want more of a good thing.

Some of you more brave souls might be asking, **"What happens when you have time left over?"** Well, to have time left over requires some skill, and also requires that you know your partner extremely well. Also, does this mean that you BOTH have time left over, or only one of the partners completes? When you both have time left over, WOW! This makes the strongest case for Six Minute Sex. Everyone feels good. Whatever the outcome, when time's left over, read chapter 3. In fact, read it anyway!

Getting together takes energy, concentration and while invigorating it is also incredibly relaxing. For some people, they might want to plan their six minute sessions, much like they would plan a date, a visit with friends or other enjoyable activity. I have heard from one friend that, every time her husband brings home a rack of lamb and a bottle of red wine, she knows it going to be a fun night. Another couple use just one word with each other - SNAP! In their lives, SNAP means Sex and a NAP! In our household, the words , "Hey, have you got six minutes?" has become almost playful foreplay, where one person clearly knows what the other is thinking. However, the children are onto us! They know all about this book. And while this is kind of cute in some ways, no child wants to envision their parents in acts of passion and intimacy.

Hugging seems to be okay, but even kissing, more than just a smooch, will have children averting their eyes and saying "ewwww!". So another phrase we use regularly is "Hey, I have an idea!"

Remember this about the spirit of six minutes, being sure those of us who have been around each other long enough for all of our warts to show, for those of us who understand that we have "bought the whole package" in terms of a partner and are happy with both the wrinkles and the bows of each other, we take the time to celebrate each other in the spirit of playfulness and curiosity.

Dr Stephen Covey, Author of 7 Habits of Highly Effective People coined the term "The Emotional Bank Account" when he was speaking of building strength in relationships. He used this phrase to **describe the level of closeness and trust, or "richness" in our relationships**. A large balance in the "bank" means lots of positive connection, trust, and closeness in the relationship. Apr. 13, 2014" Essentially Covey says, "By proactively doing things that build trust in a relationship, one makes deposits (in their partner's) Emotional Bank Account. (May 2018)"

The theory goes on to suggest that multiple deposits build a strong emotional bank account - one that is better able to sustain or withstand challenges to the relationship, to trust more deeply and to engage and celebrate each other more intimately.

So what exactly are "deposits" into the emotional bank account of our most important relationships? Lisa Gabardi (2014.04.13) offers this list:

1. Showing interest and attention
2. Offering verbal or physical affection
3. Giving compliments
4. Listening
5. Following through with commitments
6. Showing understanding
7. Apologizing
8. Showing up or spending time together are acts that offer connection, build closeness, and say *you are important to me and I value you*.

Getting Intentionally Started On Making Deposits in Your Partner's Emotional Bank Account: Using the Appreciative Approach - What are You Good At Together?

The Appreciative Approach to any situation begins with figuring out what we are good at and like doing together, and then doing more of those activities. So in your relationship, what do the two of you do together, that you like doing together, that gives you a chance to visit?   These would be things that occur during a regular day. You don't even need to be good at them, but rather recognize these as potentially positive routines that happen regularly, that you are both engaged in at the same time, where you can talk together, and build a stronger, more intimate connection. Couples that play together grow together. And if you don't grow together, you grow apart!

Some examples might include:
1. Meet for coffee in the morning, afternoon or evening
2. Visiting after work
3. Walking the dog
4. Cooking together
5. Playing card or board games or online games together
6. Cleaning the house (yes, really)
7. Taking the kids to the park/playground/forest etc
8. Shopping (food or other)
9. Outdoor work
10. Any kind of fitness activity where you can talk to each other

But be careful what you pick. Kevin and I go for bike rides which provide almost no chance to visit, as we need to ride single file for most of the way. But, we are avid skiers, and luckily ski at the same level. We visit on the chairlift up the hill, and we plan stops to connect with each other on the way down as skiing itself is a solitary sport (unless one of us falls down and can't get up after falling in deep soft snow). We have often heard one or the other of a partnership say, "Oh, I can't ski with (my partner). S/he is such a better skier than I am." I totally disagree with this. While skiing is solitary while you are skiing, there are ample opportunities to connect. Just because one partner skis green runs while the other skis something more challenging, meeting part way down or at the bottom, ensures a great recap on the way up to the top again.

We have just taken up kayaking and paddleboarding - both of which can work for talking and visiting together. We podcast together, which started out more like work, but became more fluid and natural. Although not big gamers, we like to play cards together and other traditional board games. The key is investing in the interests of each other, at least for some time interval and frequency, on a regular basis!

However, beware of seemingly great project plans and ideas that can get in the way of intimacy. Many times in our years together we have grown some wild idea that has romantic undertones, or at least that's what we thought, but have gone wrong along the way.

Boats, RV's (Recreational Vehicles) and relationships

Isn't it such a romantic idea to get a sailboat and go sailing, free in the wind, then anchor in a deserted bay off a beautiful island, dive off the bowsprit into a calm ocean? And make love to the gentle motion of the waves with no one around to hear or otherwise care? Then swim ashore and gather oysters on the beach, or dig for clams or pick muscles, put them on the barby with a big dollop of butter and garlic, all while sipping on a caesar or some cold white wine? How about gathering friends together for an afternoon sail and throwing out the crab trap? What an idyllic life, right? Well, yes… and no! How about an RV - what another fun idea! Camping on a shoreline or in the mountains, going to visit friends in other cities or towns and having your own private tiny house! Again, sounds idyllic, right? Well we have done both, and in each case, while all of those romantic and fun activities have happened for us, the part people don't talk about is the stuff that makes you wonder what you were thinking.

Take a boat. Beware of the romantic stories you hear about boats, particularly sailboats. And if you're not handy, you better be rich!! Here's the part that no one tells you about boats, and each of the points I am making are cause for a great deal of friction in your relationship. We had a sailboat - 2 in fact. What they say about boat owners? The 2 best days of your life are the day you buy your boat and the day you sell it? All true!!

1. You and your partner have to develop a special language for communicating on a boat, because when you are on deck anchoring or moving into a marina, nowhere near each other, you can't hear each other, and often can't see the other's mouth to try to make out what is being said. Hand signals are best, but if you aren't regular boaters, some signals get forgotten and mixed up and then?? Look out!!! When you end up screaming at each other, and becoming the afternoon show for others who are already anchored! Nobody wins.

2. Make sure you both have the same plans and the same goals for the investment you are making. If one isn't a fisher and the other is and thinks you are buying a fishing boat, you may not spend a lot of time together on this expensive investment, so the point is lost. If one wants to sail with the wind and the other wants to get from point A to point B, there's going to be trouble. Have an honest conversation BEFORE the purchase.

3. *Factor in the cost of the moorage for up to 5 years - then decide.*

4. *Be cautious about going into a boat partnership with a friend or friends. It sounds like the best idea you may have ever heard, to share costs and work loads, but I have heard more often that not where one partner has life changing influences, and the partnership somehow is lost.*

5. *Be prepared to have an inverse relationship that factors in fun and work, unless you are wealthy, or you love doing seasonally required boat maintenance together every year. Use a scale to rate your "fun to work" ratio. If work is your fun, then you've got it made. However, for many of us, we want to have WAY MORE fun on a boat than work we have to do on it. A "fixer upper" sounds romantic and might initially fit the budget, but beware of time and money traps. Boats take a lot of maintenance.*

6. *Be sure to USE your resource a lot more than 2 weeks a year. Otherwise rent!*
We've had much more happy success with RV's, and still going camping, both winter and summer! We seem to easily adapt to the challenges of small living spaces. But again, BEWARE!!! All big toys take maintenance, and an RV is no exception. Even purchasing an RV new will bring its headaches. Then there's storage, costly breakdowns, owning and maintaining the vehicle to tow it - can you hear the ka-ching ka-ching of the money adding up? Still, there is nothing like having all the family, and all the family pets together in a beautiful camping location with no interference. But forget the

intimacy. Until you are empty nesters and traveling as a couple, these ideas are best for building family memories!

Chapter 2

GETTING OVER THE SIX MINUTE BARRIER

No matter what, no matter where, while doing research for this book, which primarily amounted to speaking honestly and openly with strangers and friends, coworkers and bosses, gay, straight, pan, curious and undecided, even aging parents and grandparents about their intimate opportunities and habits, every single person spoken to had an intense reaction to the thought of a book on Six Minute Sex, passion and intimacy. I got the full gambit of reactions, from outrage to interest. Intense interest. But all conversations seemed to end in laughter and even more ideas. Reactions and responses have included:

Outrage (without the anger)

Six Minute Sex? That's not love, that's just sex. That can't be right.

This response came mostly from women. However, upon further conversation it became clear that for most women, they believed that they would not be able to get any satisfaction out of a six minute interlude, and therefore their time would be spent as a vessel, rather than a participant. Women want the payoff as well, but the feedback tells me that it takes longer than six minutes for many of us to go from warm to hot! Women want to cross the finish line, so to speak, and not be left hopeful and panting at the starting gate. And that is where this "idea" about intimate acts that build even more intimacy begins to take shape. Women enjoy sex just as much as men when they are equal participants, when feelings of shyness or discomfort with body changes are understood by their partner, and they are not afraid that their pleasure will be left behind. When I talk to women about ideas like "Frisky Fridays" or "Get Cracken" daybreakers, I often get such a lukewarm response. However, delving deeper into such a conversation all women agreed that, it might be true that men's and women's sex drive is more the same than different. We are both still interested, and we both want to be satisfied, and we don't want to have long sessions but we do want the benefits of how good sex makes us feel. And we want to do this with our life partner.

We also want the lasting benefits brought on by oxytocin, so that means we need to try out new routines for a period of time and then check in on the results.

If we women said to our partner, "I want us to be intimate with each other 2 times a day, every day", our partners, while perhaps being initially delighted, would likely run out of steam within a couple of days. So, somewhere between 2 times a day, 2 times a week and 2 times a month might be ideal. Increasing the frequency while decreasing the time commitment with lasting results for both parties seems to be the goal. So, make some rules, women, and know that it's brilliant to have some playfulness involved in this idea. It is meant to be fun! And safe! Say, this is going to be the "Me First" rule. It has the possibility of being sure that both partners benefit.

To get more "in the mood", women need to know how that happens for them. Perhaps prior to any action, it might help to "think it through" so to speak. For example, as a cancer survivor (or perhaps because I am just getting older and my lusty lady responses now work differently), I have discovered the amazing wonders of coconut oil and intimacy! So Simple! Even edible and good for you!

I learned that I or we could take a few minutes to read a lusty passage in a good novel. Maybe you could replay one of your top six fantasies in your mind? Think hot, alluring thoughts? Maybe you each have six minutes to get ready to begin. Taking the time to just think about how great this is going to be - how great you are going to feel, sometimes provides exactly what is needed to spark your interest. Perhaps the six minutes begins AFTER the first has reached orgasm.

But be careful! Make sure that you don't end up stalling for, and then running out of time. Maybe there are different rules for different sessions. For example, in the Follow the Leader rule, things may change depending on which partner is the leader. Whatever floats your boat - we all are sexual beings, and the benefits to spending passionate and intimate moments with the person you choose as your number 1 does nothing but good things for the both of you! And if things take longer than six minutes, who cares? No one (except perhaps you) is counting!

Curiosity -

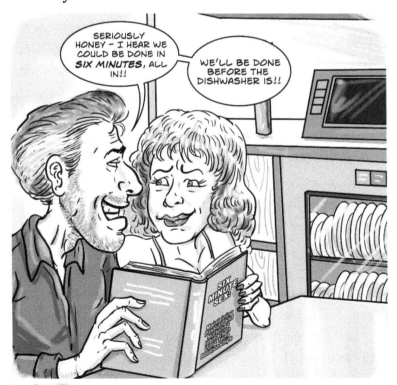

"How do you do that?"

"Can you do it in six minutes? How can you finish in six minutes?"

These responders were reminded that this was not a "How To" book, but a "Why Not?" book..

"Have you talked to my wife/husband/partner about this?"

"This is a good idea! Are you REALLY writing a book about this? I thought you were just kidding."

"What would it look like?"

All of these questions and exchanges showed me that people were curious, very curious. What would it look like if we made a lifestyle change that was an investment in each other's physical and mental well-being? What if we were proactive about our health as a couple rather than reactive and trying to repair a malaise rather than strengthen what was already healthy? The health benefits, as mentioned in the last chapter, are real. Sadly, it seems most of us are more likely to keep a commitment to a friend than one we have with our partners, or even to ourselves. So if this is indeed the case, what if we made a commitment to our partners? What if we said, "Look honey, we need to consider doing this more often. We want to be sure we are getting regular exercise, we want to keep our hearts healthy, our minds active, our love alive. We want to do whatever we can to reduce the risk of breast cancer and the risk of heart disease. We want to grow closer as we age. Here is a perfect solution, and we don't even have to leave the house, go out in the rain, drive anywhere or invite anyone else. This won't cost us much if anything, we don't need special clothes and it doesn't have to be done on anyone else's schedule but our own." Sound like a good plan?

Requests

"Can you PLEASE tell my wife about this? Don't tell her I told you to tell her. Just bring it up, like you did with me. Tell me what she says. I think it's a great idea!"

"I got a buddy who is in a rocky relationship with his wife - can you send him your manuscript? Do you think it would help?"

These responses most often came from excited husbands, and while many women might say, "well that figures...", it made me realize that our life partners still desire us. Their response, as a whole, to the idea of Six Minute Sex with their long term partners, far from being blasé, was more like "when can we get started?" What a compliment!

"When are you gonna finish this book? I know a bunch of people that would love it!"

I am delighted to say that, at no time, did anyone say "What a stupid idea", or "What a waste of time". In fact, this has been such a long project I am still surprised that friends still ask about the finish date! They are still waiting for this to be done and ready to read! I must be onto something!!

It's all about Me

"I think you should tell my story. My story lasts way longer than six minutes." This came from a beautiful looking older man who had not been able to sustain a long term intimate relationship in his adult life. Ever. He seemed more interested in sharing his multiple stories of intimacy with many partners and was perhaps trying to find a way to fit into this exclusive and elite group of long term relationship couples. However, entry to this group has extremely rigorous qualifications, and there are no exceptions. You cannot buy your way in, marry your way in, be born in or win a free pass entry. The ONLY entry is through time invested, which cannot be managed, or manufactured, hurried through or invented. Make no mistake – this is an exclusive and select group of duo's who earn their membership. Those of us that get to claim membership are proud to be a part of something this exclusive. Imagine the example we are setting for our children and our children's children.

Surprise
"You GOT to be joking! You're not? Oh, then how does that work?"
Silence

Agreement
"What a good idea! That sounds great! You better write a book about that or I will!"
But I found that some of these responders who agreed that this was a good idea were looking for, or hoping for a "how to" book. This idea of Six Minute Sex is so far from a "how to" book. There are a million books and therapists who can help us with "how to" models for those who need this kind of support.

In fact, even for those who don't think they need any "how to" ideas, a little walk on the wild side never hurt anybody, and could lead to some new, fun and worthwhile practices. Some research into this area might be more fun than they ever thought possible. However, this author is not an expert on sex. My motivation is a strong belief, well supported by research, that intimacy builds strong relationships, more laughter and longer lives!

"Why would you want to do that?"

Well, why not?

This, I believe, translated into "please don't give him any more ideas", and what a shame that is to hear. Reluctant partners, please think about this. After a very long time together, it is incredibly flattering to know that your long term partner still has the hots for you. You STILL make him or her turn around, stop and stare, and that person STILL wants to be intimate with you. That person STILL wants to jump your bones. WOW! That has got to be the most amazing compliment in the world. Take advantage of it, revel in it, enjoy it. Because for too many of us, if we suddenly ended up alone after a very long time, we likely would want to know that we spent our very best years together with our very best number 1 person, engaged in deep and loving intimacy. We will have memories which we will cherish forever. And while it likely won't be the six minute interludes that we will daydream about, our warm and loving memories will be enhanced by the intimacy we experienced together in our daily lives. Our deep feelings for each other; the way we integrated with each other; our ability to communicate with no words; these memories will help sustain us through the loss. This is what we will stare off into sunsets remembering.

The Challenge of Intimacy: Where does the time go?

Without exception, time and timing seem to be one of the biggest challenges to maintaining regular intimate opportunities. Well, time and place together. Why is that? As often happens, time goes by and then one morning we look at each other and think, "when was the last time we…." and realize it's been like a desert around the house in terms of intimacy. I get cranky. I now know that if I am getting cranky and have little patience with things and people, intimacy has been lacking. Other times, somehow we just seem to put everything else before ourselves and each other, and when we finally get around to investing some time, we look at each other afterward and say something like, "God, why don't we do that more often?"

In fact, as we spend more and more time with one another we become a part of one anothers' rhythms of life. As we age together, we get more comfortable with just being around each other. We may even take advantage of the fact that our partner is always around and that the good stuff, like intimacy, can happen any time, which usually translates into "later".

But ask any widower what they would be willing to give for just one more day, one more lunch, even just a few more minutes with their life partner. Their first wish would likely not be to engage in a physically intimate act, but rather to bask in the afterglow of such an investment and spend time loving and visiting. More often than not, a widowed partner would willingly give their own life in trade for their spouse's. But trades cannot happen and we cannot change what is done. Therefore, leave no opportunity for regrets or "if only's". The time to act is now, not later. Not when the babies are kids or the kids are grown ups or tomorrow. Not when the dishes are done, or the laundry is on or the groceries are put away. Not when you've finished your email or paid the bills online. Because if you wait to be finished you will wait forever. There is no finishing of the dishes, the laundry, the email, the bills or any other life tasks. Lifetimes are journeys of repetition and new experiences. The repetitions get in the way of the new experiences sometimes. There really is no tomorrow with the promise of more free time.

My daughter reminds me, in other conversations, that tomorrow never comes. Nothing could be more true of an opportunity lost. Think of that the very next time the person you chose to spend the rest of your life with wants to jump your bones. What a compliment! Take the time. You'll never regret it.

Chapter 3

WHAT HAPPENS WHEN YOU HAVE TIME LEFT OVER?

Old people's sex is different than young people's sex. Especially old people's sex who are in long term monogamous relationships. Who would disagree? Sex and intimacy for us long term relationship people, while certainly connected and related, are not necessarily co-dependent. You can have one without the other. They are closely intertwined, and BOTH, together or separate, can provide us with deep feelings of gratitude and love for the other. It is the intimate connection that provides the greatest payoff. Sex and intimacy have the same benefits and keep us younger longer.

Having said that, any couple who has time left over has clearly been thinking about this for some time. There is ANTICIPATION, knowing what's coming soon. There's EXCITEMENT thinking about the when and the how! There's the PREPARATION: get naked (or not), think steamy - replay in your mind a past great session and get ready. STOP thinking about today's to-do list or yesterday's frustrations. Think only of your partner and what's coming! Anticipate success. And there's a THRILL when the plan is followed through. You have to know each other extremely well in order to have time left over. You have to be focussed on the task rather than the time! And you have to be OK with changing your routine of intimacy.

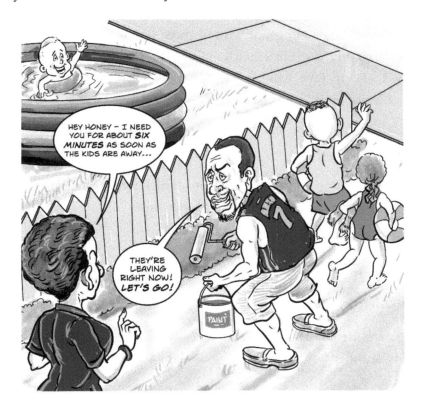

"Time left over?" you ask. "How is that possible"

"That's impossible"

"They're lying"

Well, all I can say is that it is not impossible, and that couples have been known to arrive at the finish line before the six minute is up, happy and healthy, albeit a little out of breath. And what the rest of us have to say to that is Bravo and Well Done! Keeping in mind that this is not ever intended to be a race to the finish, when two people can be involved intimately and both parties be mutually satisfied in less than six minutes, it means a lot of things, and all of them good. It's not a goal, but rather an idea. Let's face it, no one is interested in the book called "Forty Five Minute Sex: What Happens When You Have Time Left Over?"

So, when this raging phenomenon occurs, what then????

Brag to each other

Try to figure out all of the conditions which made that possible so you can recreate them again another time

Find your clothes

Rush off to work with a smile on your face

Smooth the bed

Pour a coffee, a glass of wine, mix a martini, crack a beer or enjoy another kind of refreshing beverage

Sit and just smile to yourself and your partner

Go back to whatever you were doing without much disruption such as: losing the internet connection; the water boiling over; the garlic burning; the kids noticing

Rest

Relax

Whatever you want!

Because the option is, what would you rather not do?? If you took advantage of six minutes with your partner, here's what you wouldn't have to do!

Drag yourself out of bed

Set a special time and place to exercise

Launder your exercise clothes

Use anti- wrinkle cream that day

Worry about not being active enough

Feel guilty

Wonder when the next rendezvous would be

Avoid

Avoiding means you are thinking about it, but you are hoping it doesn't come up. It might be interesting to consider the reasons behind avoiding. Is there a shyness with body changes creeping in? Does it just feel like too much work? Has there been a change in your life pattern that one partner is not adapting to? Is one partner mad at the other? Did something happen that rocked one's world and not the others?

Kevin and I were together for many years before we got married. In fact, when I first met Kevin, he told me that he was NEVER getting married and NEVER having kids. For me, he was just a cute nice guy when we met - I couldn't care less if he planned to marry and have kids or not. I was just coming out of a short term marriage and not at all interested in doing that again any time soon. But time went by and we stayed together, and naturally people started asking us out loud about our long term plans. The truth was, for a long time, we had no long term plans. And we were together for such a long time with no engagement in sight, people finally stopped asking. So 6 years into it, we made a five year plan with a firm date set, and no one believed that we were ever going to get hitched. But we did -July 3, 1993 was our special day. But it almost didn't happen!

It's crazy what comes by to try us and challenge us on our most personal level, but this was a show stopper for us, and nearly a deal breaker. My most wonderful auntie died late 1992. She was an artist, and had been a caregiver to me and my siblings when we were children. Even though she looked after us at our house from Monday to Friday, while both my parents worked full time, we would go to her house on a Sunday afternoon and she would have us baking cakes and cookies, painting and pastelling - being creative and loving it. She never minded the mess we would get into, and she was as selfless a person who ever lived. She fed our minds and our imaginations, and her love had no boundaries!! So, I wanted Kevin and I to attend her funeral. He refused. Told me to go myself. I couldn't believe it. Although he didn't know her, he knew what she meant to me. But he would not go. So, to shrink a long story, I told him that we needed to get some help because this was a big deal for me, and I didn't want to carry on with the wedding plans until we untangled what was wrong in our relationship. While Kevin initially was reluctant, we did pursue counseling therapy, both as a couple and as individuals. Kevin said he couldn't understand why I thought we needed counseling therapy- after all, we had about the best relationship of all the friends we knew. Couples who were friends of ours had met, married, had children and divorced in the same timeline that we had been together. We were both devastated to think that we might not make it. But there was something fundamentally wrong, and I insisted we explore.

We worked with a gifted counselor. At one point she asked each of us, separately, what we would do if we were not able to resolve the issue. We both said that the relationship would have to end. But neither of us wanted that, so we worked REALLY HARD to fix our own behaviors that triggered the other - to better understand how to stand together stronger, and in love - to not compromise the other in any way. She helped us change, grow, adapt and move forward with a strong commitment to each other, and a common vision for the future. And we never looked back. The wedding went forward. I learned to stop pushing so hard when I wanted something, he learned not to check out emotionally and stop sitting on the fence. The work we did then has helped us through so many hard times - times that may have broken other relationships but rather strengthened ours. It was the best investment we ever made - in ourselves and each other!

Sometimes disagreements and/or situations happen that, without resolution, could leave a lasting scar on the relationship. The story above describes an impasse that we came to and, for some reason, could not get over, through, around or otherwise get by without some professional help. Along the journey to understanding and resolution, we were able to smooth over many bumps we didn't even know existed, which both of us ultimately believe strengthened our foundation and allowed our intimate connection to bond even more deeply. So our feelings of care for each other, for protecting one another, for sheltering each other from the pain of life's extreme challenges runs deep, and we do good things for ourselves and each other that seem like an investment in wellness.

So…..

The What If's?

What if? you and your partner were guaranteed a better chance to have a healthy heart by engaging in regular acts of intimacy together?

What if? you were given a free card for reducing your chances of contracting breast cancer if you committed to having regular intimate acts with your partner?

What if? you were promised happiness that could withstand some of life's toughest challenges that inevitably come our way that would make you and your partner stronger?

What if? the two of you were guaranteed to grow closer and closer emotionally, spiritually and in every other way if you just committed to enjoying each other regularly without interference?

What if? your kids were both embarrassed and proud that their parents still flirted with each other?

What if? younger couples pointed you out to each other when they see you walking down the street holding hands, hoping that someday that would be them?

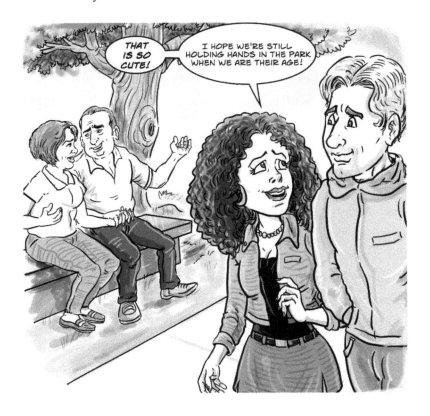

What if ? this is just a good idea all around?

What if...

Of course there are no guarantees in life and we have to go by what we believe. But how many times have you seen the following scenario, or perhaps even lived it yourself.

You and your partner are living life just fine thank you very much. You are busy with friends and family, reasonably successful in all aspects of life, your kids are well, you enjoy what you are doing and you are cruising through life, however you and your partner have grown physically and/or emotionally apart from each other, and you don't make the time to be together in an intimate way. Then, one day, one of you finds out about a health issue that, while risky, can be managed through diet, exercise and positive outlooks. Suddenly you both REACT to that threat. Lifestyles change immediately. Diets change, routines change and you find yourselves fighting for your life together. The reaction to the threat is significant. Well, what if regular acts of intimate, loving, mutually satisfying sex and other intimate acts helps to build a barrier against bad things so that you may never find yourselves in that position? Would that be worth it? Too often we find ourselves being reactive rather than proactive. We stop doing what we know can harm us once the harm has begun! Taking care of ourselves and each other, loving ourselves and each other, and making time for intimacy and passion enhances every aspect of a healthy life. Don't wait for problems to present themselves. Put yourselves FIRST on your "to do " list.

Remember that this book is not a "how to" book, but rather a "why wouldn't you?" book. The message here is that, as we age and grow more and more familiar with each other, we begin to take for granted the person that is always there, that we expect will always be there. For the most part, we already have long days and full lives, and let's face it, to refrain from doing one more thing that is absolutely not necessary is so tempting. Intimacy takes time and energy. And sometimes patience. It takes desire and focus. And it also takes passion and will. With our ever busy lives, it just seems easier to put off the "pay off" tasks and take the easier road. After all, so many things we do each day require us to take the harder road, or the higher road, or the road that requires energy and patience. Besides that, there is no life threatening condition that I know of that requires us to engage in passionate pleasures in order to stay alive. By that I mean that making love with our partner is not the antidote for a life threatening disease, but it may be a preventative measure. And while we all know that exercise is good for us, it's more of an insurance policy than a magic pill. So I encourage you to listen to that little voice inside you - the one that preserves, not the one that sabotages. We all have both voices operating inside of us, and we can use them to our advantage. As well, and perhaps surprisingly, sometimes those people closest to us can help guide us to make decisions that enhance our lives, and perhaps even keep us safe! So be sure to listen to your own inside self, and to others who know and love you, when they "get a feeling" about something.

Here's a story for you about that little voice - remember that people who really know you and love you hear little voices too - and sometimes the message is worth listening to.

My mom seemed to have a gift of seeing certain things before they happened. As weird as it sounds, she seemed to see, in her dreams, births and deaths somehow related to those closest to her, and her circle of friends knew of this gift and saw it in action many times. When she had a dream that her best friend was going to get hit by a car and killed, she called her and told her about the dream. Two weeks later mom's friend called to thank her for the warning - sure enough she was about to step out to cross the street, remembered my mom's warning (they had a long long friendship) so she stopped when she otherwise likely would not have, and narrowly escaped being "plowed over" by a fast moving vehicle. As well, my mom had a dream about our next door neighbor having another child. She already had 5 children and she had her hands full, and when my mom said, "Kaye, I had a dream you were pregnant," our next door neighbor said "I don't think so", but 6 weeks later she confirmed the healthy pregnancy!

So, fast forward to my adult life. I inherited none of this gift, but my siblings may have. One year I decided to ride my bike to work everyday in an attempt to get fit and save some money. My siblings knew of my effort, so when the phone rang at 5:30 one morning with a sister on the line, asking if I was going to ride to work that day, I said yes. She said - DON'T. I saw you in a dream get hit and killed at the intersection at the top of your street. So, that day, I didn't ride my bike. But 6 weeks later when my brother called me at 6:00 in the morning with the same story, I never rode my bike to work again that year. I trusted that the people who love me had some kind of warning signal that I didn't have, and I respected that. I didn't want to test out the accuracy of their messages, because - what if they were right? *Anyway, why the story? Because people who love us try to protect us. Never dismiss the power of love.*

No Regrets - You've Heard This Before

Remember when you couldn't keep your hands off each other? When your thoughts were occupied with how much longer you had to wait until you could be together? It wasn't so long ago. Remember how much fun it was. Over time, our desire to be intimate with one another grows if we tend to it. Like anything we take pride in, our intimate relationships are fueled by a passion, and flourish like a well tended garden with time and care and practice. When we pursue intimacy regularly, our shared love for and commitment to each other strengthens, with each partner taking the lead at different times!

But just imagine if that lovely, important, caring warm body was not there every day. What if something happened? What would be your regrets? What would you wish you had done more of? Tasks and jobs? Cutting the lawn or painting the family room? Really, if tragedy struck, your memories would likely be with your intimate moments, your fun times, and your shared secrets, and you might be willing to make any bargain to get one more chance. We need to live our lives with no regrets, and this is just one example of how we can do that.

As a reminder, this is a book intended for those of us in long term intimate relationships, lifelong commitments. There is a story that goes something like this:

> If a couple, upon meeting, falling and in love and becoming intimate, were to put coin in a jar every time there made love for the first 18 months, they would surely amass a great number of coins. The challenge then switches itself around. So, if that same couple were to stay together and after the initial 18 months, they should REMOVE a coin for every time they are intimate, they would die without having emptied the jar!

While there may be some truth to that story, the fact is that for most of us in long term relationships, that water just doesn't get hotter as time goes by. USA Today (Feb. 2020) says that for optimum health, we should be making love with our partners at least once a week. At least! Sounds tiring just reading that, don't you think? However, we need to update our lovemaking strategies and methods of lovemaking from our youth. If we can switch our thinking around and invite some whimsy into this idea, then intimacy begins to sound a little naughty and a little bit more like fun rather than a chore. Put aside past, predetermined practices. Intimacy doesn't have to follow a pre-set pattern. Six minutes (or less) of sex can fit into the tightest of schedules! Remember back to the days of young love and the magic of 6 minute sex, when it was either in play or at least on our minds EVERY six minutes? And it usually lasted much longer than 6 minutes! Time to update our strategies!

So let's talk about the routine of intimacy. We all have our own rhythms, whether it's circadian, diurnal, ultradian, infradian or something else, as we all age, we begin to notice that our desires for certain things occur most strongly at certain times of the day. Sleep, food, company, and intimacy. And it gets a bit tricky if each partner feels most amorous at a different time of the day (or night). Are mornings best? Afternoons? Evenings? Is one partner on shift work? Do your weeks have different work days? Well, no one said this was going to be easy, and besides, you know each other well enough to get around those details! But you have to **want** to get around the details, because, as you may have noticed, there is ALWAYS a reason not to!

Some couples tell me that sometimes the rush and anticipation leaves them with some of their clothes still on. One couple reports back, "Cindy, we just can't do it in six minutes. Eight minutes is the best it gets!" another couple reports - "About 12 minutes is best for both of us, ya about 12 minutes". These folks are having fun with this idea. They are not letting routine get in the way of whimsy and playfulness. And heaven knows we can all do with a little more playfulness.

So what happens when you have time left over ? WHOO-HOO is what I have to say! Well done and high five! While it seems impossible, this question has come up. Laugh if you will, or let your head go wherever it goes when it is trying to process and assimilate something that just doesn't seem possible, it is indeed possible to be fully satisfied, yes BOTH of you fully satisfied, and have a bit of time left over. When that happens, you should brag about it, even if just with each other. Another benefit to think about is this - if it only takes us a few minutes, maybe we could do it more often?

Six Minute Sex with mutual satisfaction in 4 minutes (or 5 minutes and 59 seconds) is quite an accomplishment. It means that you and your partner know each other REALLY well. It means that you have both been anticipating this time together and you've already started before you've even started. It means that, like the old "mile high" club, you have bragging rights! "Sooner than Six" raises eyebrows and egos, not to mention feeling pretty good about being able to satisfy your partner faster than you can bring water to a boil. It is a rare occurrence for most of us, but it happens and we don't seem to forget it.

But remember, this is not really a race. This is not a competition, nor is it a test. It is an idea, an idea that is a little bit fun, a little bit "out of the box" and a little bit naughty. Because in order to talk about it, the Six Minute Sex thing, in order to talk about it past the idea stage, you have to be willing to try it. And being willing to try it, even if you are long past your 40's, means that you still have a sense of whimsy about sex, and that you know that every time you make love with your partner, it does not have to be like a recommitment to your life together, or a zen-like experience. It does not need to be that intense. It can just be a "quicky".

Fast and fun.

Clumsy.

Partially clothed, standing, sitting, leaned over, or lying down or ??

On the bed or off the bed.

Choose a room.

Surprise one another. You are unlikely to regret it.

It can be in the walk-in closet (so I'm told - I don't have one), the regular closet (although, why would you?), the bathroom, the basement, the attic, and yes, even the bedroom. Some say that it can be in the car. Not so much for us, the car.

It can be six or sixty minutes, or 4 or 40 minutes.

The benefits are the same. The memories still linger and your skin glows. Your heart is happy, and you get a bit of a workout. It counts.

Maybe it is the magic pill!!!

But the ultimate goal is to maintain passion and nurture intimacy.

The six minute dash is kind of a fun idea, and quite honestly, if you are spending six minutes completely focused on you and your partner, how bad can that be?

Don't wait until the end of the day. Then you might just decide to wait until tomorrow morning because you are too tired. Then you sleep in and then you wait again until the end of the day. This "OK, Later, OK, Later" cycle is off putting, makes it seem like we are not interested in each other, and lulls our sensuous senses into flat boredom.

Don't wait until the kids are in bed, then for sure you'll be too tired. Kids seem to have this sense that something special is coming, and on those nights that have been so carefully planned by you, everything goes out the window when the baby fusses or the little ones just won't go down. TAKE ADVANTAGE of those moments when the baby falls asleep in the swing. I can almost guarantee you that the child will sleep for at least six minutes. Be close enough to hear the baby wake up, but far enough away that you feel like the two of you are on your own.

In the fabulous Walt Disney movie," The Emperor's New Groove", one scene shows the kids so excited with the return of their father that they just will not go to bed. Dad finally comes up with a brilliant idea and says to the kids, "Well, that just fine if you want to stay up with us. Your mom and I are just going to be smooching on the couch!" and he kisses her cheek. Well both the kids say , "EWWWW" and off to bed they go.

That's Brilliant! And who said Disney is just for kids?

Try it. It works. I know because I've used that strategy many times, and each time we get the same reaction "EWWWWW!"

Chapter 4

WHAT HAPPENS WHEN SIX MINUTES IS NOT ENOUGH?

What Six minute Sex Is	What Six Minute Sex Isn't
An opportunity	A dumb Idea
Fun	Impossible
A gift	Just sex*
Good connection time	A race
Enjoyable	Another task
Creative	Not worth it
Worth it!	A promise of good health, it IS, however, a preventative measure
A chance to deepen the bond	A chore
An investment in good health	A waste of time

*sometimes it is just sex, which is fun too

What a strange and interesting question, you might be saying to yourself. "Of course six minutes is not enough time," you might be thinking. "That's ridiculous!" Six Minute Sex might feel, at first suggestion, a crazy stupid idea. But it grows on people and mostly, it brings a smile to the faces of those with imagination. Six Minute Sex is meant to be seen as an opportunity to build the relationship with your life partner even closer and more intimate. After peeling back the layers of this inviting and inventive idea, the six minutes part ceases to be the most important.

The key to this is finding intimate time with each other. Keep in mind that there are no hard and fast rules. Six Minute Sex does not have to be sex, but you do want to be engaging in some kind of intimate behaviour together regularly. Six Minute Sex is not a race, unless you want it to be one. This is not a threat, which sounds coercive and mean spirited. This is not a command as in "thou shalt...". This is a gift, a lucky idea, a fantasy come true. This is not a dumb idea. This is meant to be fun and enjoyable. You are not on a time clock, except the timer that you put yourselves on. No one wants to know "how did it go?", or "did you make it". No one is gathering data or comparing some against others. Six minutes is a fun idea, and should bring a smile to your face. Take all the time you like. Just be sure to take the time. Sometimes we are both so tired at night that we think it is just good enough that we are interested in each other and talking about it, even if the "main event" does not happen. As we have aged, our "Frisky Fridays" have sometimes evolved to "it counts if you think about it!" as our eyes slam shut with our heads on the pillow!

Remember that this idea is intended to bring long-timers together and rekindle the passion, as well as to add a pretty big dose of whimsy back into your intimate lives. During the research I did for the book, one couple kept telling me, "Cindy, anything over 8 minutes will work for us. That's our best. As for six minutes? Nope!"

 We just can't make it happen in six minutes!" another couple reported, "all we have ever needed is 7 minutes! That's the way it's always been with us!" Both couples were having some fun with this notion of six minutes.   They were enjoying themselves and each other, and most important, they were doing it together.

And it is high time that we long loving couples claim our special and important place in the 21st Century, and celebrate our mutual survival of COVID, with our passion for each other mostly intact. That was a terribly hard 2 plus years, and we will be feeling the negative effects, I believe, for years to come. But it cautiously feels like we are on the other side of the pandemic.

We become the role models for our grown kids and others who know of our commitment to each other, and for surviving a hard patch. We set the stage for what our children can expect as they age with their chosen partners, even when faced with a pandemic. We are their model, and those who choose to invest in their shared intimacy provide their kids with a bullet proof formula for maintaining passion and nurturing intimacy up to and fully including old age. When life is all rushing around, moving faster and more efficiently, every new thing looks shiny and important. Change is thrown at us daily, and for some of us in the second half of our lives, the learning curve to manage daily life is pretty steep. But with intimacy, and the time we have invested in our intimate past, we pave the way for an exciting intimate future.

Do you know that, our youngsters, when they get married, they brag about us?? They talk about us when we are not around in ways that let us know they've noticed. Young couples getting married say, "well my parents have been together for 35 years, and you know what, they still do it!" and they say it in a way that makes them proud, while scrunching their faces to show their displeasure at knowing about intimacy and its importance in our lives.

So, what qualifies as a life partner? Many of us are not in our first committed relationship, but still consider the relationship we are in as our lifetime commitment. This may not be your first or second partner, but this IS your life partner. What does it take to be a lifer? Well, look at the list below and see if anything fits!

1. You must have been together for what YOU define as a lifetime together

2. All things being equal, you must look quite a bit different now than you did when you met

3. When you first got together, TV was popular and commercials came on every 12 or so minutes

4. Again, when you first met, likely cell phones were still a bit of a novelty, or perhaps didn't even exist. No one under the age of 10 owned one.

Does that make some sense? Does that sound like you and your partner? Because those of us that got out of abusive relationships, that moved past the hurting and found someone to feed our souls (and vice versa), those of us who were widowed and heartbroken but able to move on and find someone else who really loves us, those of us who have had to leave relationships and move on to find someone who refreshes us rather than wears us out, or those who lost in love but moved on and found their life partner - we are all lifers! To get into this club takes years - that's really the only criteria besides being committed to each other. That, and you likely relate to many of the stories told in this book!

But we must avoid the trap of living together like brother and sister, and here's the reason. While friendship with your partner is most important, it is even more important to have a circle of friends that does not always include your lifemate. You can have as many friends as your time permits, as your heart can hold, as your life can manage, but you only get one long-time lifemate (at a time!). That person has a special and most important role in your life. Be sure that you do not confuse the roles and responsibilities of your intimate life partner with others who also matter deeply, but differently to you.

It may be helpful if we can broaden our definition of what equals intimacy, as intimacy does not necessarily mean sex. For some couples, the idea of getting naked and then being intimate seems overwhelming, especially if this has not really been the practice for such a long time. Intimacy can take many forms and does not have to be limited by any means by preconceived ideas.   If you are looking for ways to spend six minutes that count as intimate, consider the following:

Start Slow

Go for a walk and hold hands (usually takes longer than six minutes, but remember the name of the chapter).

How lovely is it to see a more mature couple holding hands as they stroll along? Do we all automatically think that they must be in a new relationship? YES!! But isn't it great when we find out they are lifers - still interested enough in each other in that romantic way that they want to hold hands? So, so charming!

Sit close enough to each other so that your legs are touching. Feel the heat of the other's body and touch.

Stand really close to one another and look straight into each other's eyes.

Compliment one another, not on a special occasion, but just because.

Perform an act of kindness that is intended to surprise the other. See what happens.

Warm it up a bit

Kiss, and I mean kiss. Not a peck, not a smooch but a kiss. Not a duty kiss or a patterned kiss, like the ones you might have when you part, or when you see each other, or even when you go to bed each night. I mean KISS! I think we used to call it necking, however that term came to be! If the other partner starts the kiss, make sure you do it back.

Hold each other in bed – a full frontal hold. Hang onto one another for a while and don't let go. Rub your partner's back. This "hug" needs to last at least 20 seconds to have good mental and physical health benefits.

Read a sexy romantic book together, in bed or anywhere.

Watch a movie rated "R", and don't try to pretend it has no effect on you! It's SUPPOSED to have an effect on you!

Play a game called "the most romantic time we have had together".

Retell your "when we first met" stories to each other.

Dance together a slow dance, anywhere, when an old favorite comes on. We sometimes dance in the short little hallway in our 17 foot trailer. It's ALWAYS my idea, but he is ok with that. We always kiss at the end, and I know that he doesn't always enjoy kissing, but he knows that I do!

If you just don't dance, take a class for some kind of dancing that requires you to hold each other close! Practise at home, on the deck, in the trailer, in the kitchen before dinner!

Buy champagne, chill the glasses and put on some music and see what happens!

Hot

Plan a date night (see chapter six. Check the **Order of Operations** for date night. **Spoiler alert: It says, Make sure you have sex first**)

Choose to spend some intimate time together.

Sleep naked.

Put on something that makes you smell good.

Dress up for your partner as a surprise.

Buy your partner some fundies - fun and sexy underwear!

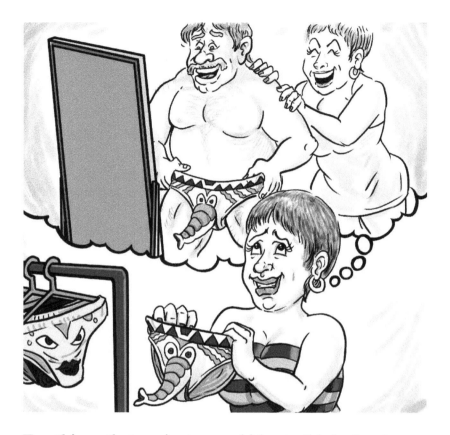

Ten things that are just a good idea to think about

1.   Get rid of the TV in the bedroom
2.   Shut the pets OUT of the room once in a while
3.   If you have little kids, have a lock on the top inside of your bedroom door. If they try to get in at an inconvenient time, pretend that there was a sock stuck under the door. Don't forget to take the lock off after a rendezvous if it is late at night.
4.   Turn the ringer off, do not leave on the vibrate.

5. Check the alarm BEFORE!
6. Drunk sex is never really good sex, even if it seems like it MIGHT be a good idea at the time. Although it is super fun and still worth a shot, it often goes on for hours, no one gets to the finish line, and it leaves a rash - and the reason I know this is because... still, don't completely dismiss the idea!
7. Don't eat in bed.
8. Lit candles are dangerous! Use the battery operated ones.
9. Preserve the time for each other.
10. Choose your time and stick to it – don't let anything (barring emergencies) interfere.

6 more great reasons for considering this option

1. Because you CAN!
2. Because you will both feel better and you will live longer.
3. Because you don't need a special outfit (although you might want one), you don't need special shoes, you don't need to drive anywhere, you don't need to be on a set schedule.
4. Because you will be showing your children, your relatives, your friends and anyone else who happens to be around you that, after all this time, it still matters to you both.
5. Because you CAN! (Did I say that already?) and finally...
6. Because we will not live forever - no one gets out of this life alive and we cannot predict what the future holds!

I spent a number of years in my adult life being overweight. Not just a little, but a lot. Throughout all of this time, my husband not only loved me, he desired me. He seemed invisible to the extra weight and was my biggest fan forever. It was me who had the problem with my weight, and as a result, I think my feelings made us miss out on many intimate opportunities. The lesson? When we are truly with our life partner, it is literally through thick and thin. Excuses are lame. Redefine intimacy if you must, but grab some serious loving time together.

Well when six minutes is simply not enough, that's great. Remember that the slogan "Six Minutes" is a metaphor for "Why wouldn't we?" It really isn't the timing that matters, it is the TAKING TIME that matters. Six minutes seems a little ridiculous for many people. For some of us, it takes at least that much time to shed our clothes (really?). Some start the timing from the moment that the idea is born. If you happen to be out shopping, well, forget about the timer. Anticipation is an aphrodisiac, and in such cases, it's worth the wait.

Other things that take six minutes and aren't nearly as good for you:

Unloading the dishwasher

Mashing potatoes

Switching laundry loads and folding

Making a grilled cheese sandwich

Switching cars

Recalling an incident from the day

Disagreeing with who was supposed to pick up the prescription

Loading the car

Unloading the car

Looking for the keys (just get the spare set)

Responding to email

Downloading music

Making lunches

Dog play

Editing your child's essay on Peace

Cleaning the stain on the carpet

Boiling water

Changing the sheets

Washing the kitchen floor

Organizing the junk drawer in the kitchen

The Sad Side of This Idea

Some couples think that the idea of Six Minute Sex is cheap, and it cheapens sex to the point of, well, just being sex. I say that cheap sex is better than no sex.

I love to hear of couples that take the time for intimacy with each other A LOT AND OFTEN. I remember an old acquaintance telling me that, after she and her husband had an intimate rendezvous, he would be so much more attentive and affectionate. More "touchy", really, which kept her interest in being intimate alive and active. I think that for her, those extra hours of affection were just as important to her. I also think that their physical investment in each other paid off in many residual ways.

And it is so important for our children to see us being playful with each other. When I was a kid, if we saw our parents embrace or even kiss it was unusual, so readers can understand what a shocking surprise it was for me and one of my sisters when we witnessed our dad gently tug the towel off of our mom as she made the dash from the shower to their bedroom. He clearly had no idea that we were there! We were SHOCKED (but not as shocked as my mom was when she heard the two of us gasp), and she gently scolded my dad. He just giggled, but it introduced to us a playfulness between them that we seldom witnessed. It made us feel happy and I think secure, seeing our parents at play. So I encourage you to be a model of whimsy for your kids, now and again, so they see that the two of you still have some "teenage fun", even after years of being together!

One evening, Kevin and I decided to have a hot tub. With the layout of our home, our bedrooms are on the bottom floor, along with the family room and a couple of bathrooms. In order to reach the outside hot tub from our bedroom, we have to walk past the outside of the family room windows. And because we really have a private backyard, we often just wrap towels around ourselves on our journey to and from the hot tub, especially in the dark. On this particular evening, I was feeling quite playful, and as we made our way back to our bedroom, I noticed that both our daughters were in there

watching TV . I said to Kevin "Let's flash them!" Well, Kevin would
no sooner flash anyone (let alone his daughters) than he would fly to
the moon, but I was game. Anyway, I knocked on the window to get
their attention, we turned our backs to them and I dropped my towel!
Kevin just kind of wiggled his bum with his towel on. Both of the
girls said "ewwwwh" and looked at each other. One said to the other,
"What is wrong with our parents?". We laughed and laughed - a
great example of our kids seeing their old parents being playful. And
when I think about some of the tough times we have come through, I
am so grateful that our girls have seen us manage the good, the bad
and the ugly!!

I think it's fantastic when I meet and talk to long term relationship couples who still can't keep their hands off each other. Wow. I think that, from time to time, I am mostly just jealous! The thing is, I so rarely meet those couples, and I talk to a lot of people about this topic.

Some of the secrets that have been shared with me!

Look into the eyes of the person you have chosen, and who chose you all those years ago. Remember getting lost in those eyes. Look again- like you used to. Shut everything else out. Remember thinking how beautiful those eyes are. Remember swimming in them. Swim again! Don't talk. Gently touch the face of your beloved. Smile at your chosen. Be still. Say "I love you". See what happens.

Reach out and hug. Or say, "come here for a minute," and open your arms. Hug generously with as much frontal contact as possible. This is your partner, not your companion. Remember to hold onto that full body hug for at least 20 seconds. Whisper something loving into the ear of your partner. Inhale. Exhale. See what happens.

Choose your timing wisely. Make sure no deadlines are approaching, no kids are about to come in the door. Turn your phone off first. Setting a surprisingly loving and intimate mood on a whim can lead to many good things. Remember that YOU determine the parameters and set the mood. Don't wait for the opportunity to be presented to you, present it yourself. You are the driver in this relationship just as much as your partner is, and the invitation to intimacy is an elixir!

Six minutes, four minutes, 12 minutes - it just doesn't matter. What matters is that you take the time with each other for intimacy. You can set aside a whole evening or just a "coffee break". Regret seems like so much energy expended for no good reason.

And as a sidenote, for most of us who have not maintained that level of connection over the many years of commitment and companionship, intimacy does not mean just sex and orgasm, or just racing to the finish line. Enjoying each other privately through talking, touching, hand holding, snuggling, massaging, good back scratches foot rubs - any intimate act really, keeps us close emotionally. My friend Jill just asked me the other day, "Why do foot rubs always end up with sex?" We both laughed! By adjusting our expectations for intimacy when we need to, and "updating" those expectations from our early years we can make plans that are much more practical and realistic. The journey at our age is perhaps just as good and satisfying as reaching the finish line!

Chapter 5

WHAT'S THE SECRET TO SUCCESS?

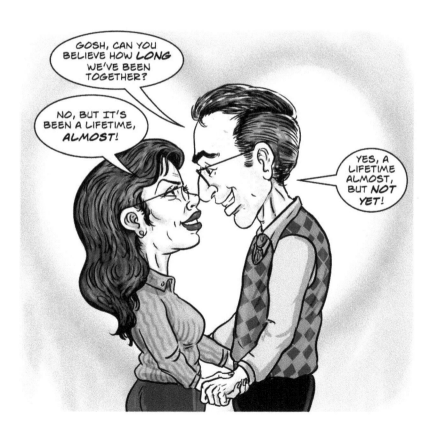

Chapter 5 is a little different than the other chapters. As I try to sort out the chronological order of events and stories, given the time lapse between the start and the finish of this book, I have struggled with how to present this chapter of stories and information. What makes the most sense is to date the stories and updates to the stories, not necessarily in chronological order, but to provide a way for readers to process the information and build on prior knowledge. My goal of course is that all of this makes sense to readers because this is important information. This chapter was meant to provide the secret as to how to stay together and in love after over 30 years together. I started by interviewing couples who had been together for over 30 years, now I am a part of a couple who have been together for over 30 years! So time has certainly slipped by! Anyway…

Summer 2010 - Thanks to Jane, who first suggested it, and Joanne at Yellow Point Lodge who gave me the idea that this book on Six Minute Sex needed to have a chapter on relationships, or more pointedly, on relationships that have survived, how they have survived, what it took to survive, and what makes them keep on ticking. I wrote this introduction prior to doing the work that needs to be done to complete this chapter because I have some ideas about what I am going to learn. You see, this chapter will be composed of interviews with couples who have been together 30 plus years, and what they think the magic is.

When the idea for Chapter 5 first presented itself, I was floating on the ocean with two other kayaks. One of the kayaks had me and my husband in it, one had our friends Jane and Ian, and the other, the kayak in the middle or our flotilla, had Brad in it. You see, Brad was on his own because he had just recently lost the love of his life, his beloved Barb. He lost her to breast cancer, and the two of them had fought that hideous disease to the last. They had fought it together with love and laughter and life, rather than bitterness and anger and sadness.

Now that was a match made in heaven. Brad and Barb were such a great couple, they were a favorite of all of us. These two celebrated life in BIG ways, always with fun and great storytelling, and those of us lucky enough to bask in their light had a better life because of it.

Even before Barb was diagnosed with terminal cancer, the two of them enjoyed every moment of being together. They sailed, they camped, they traveled, they belonged to the MG club and went on weekend excursions. They planned and played and celebrated every moment of life, and they shared this celebration with everyone around them. And even though they had each been married to another before they began their journey together, they managed to spend 30 years totally devoted to each other.

Out on the ocean, we had the honor of being with Brad as he said one of his farewells to Barb. He lifted a container and let the wind spread some of Barb's ashes before us. We gently dropped flowers into the ocean, watching the myriad of colors spread in a carpet around us. And we raised our glasses together as we sipped on a champagne toast to our friend Barb, right out there on the ocean.

Tears were shed. Not a lot, but those quiet gentle tears of love and loss slipped down our cheeks and found a resting place on our shirt collars. It was a moment in life, grand and sad all at one time.

Then we started to talk as we drifted. We reminisced about our friend and how much she loved where we were. We talked about Barb and Brad's passion for each other and for their life together. We remembered how they reveled in each other's company and the company of their friends. And that's when it happened. Jane said, in her fabulous Welsh accent, "Well Cindy, you must write about them. This is your chapter 5. You must write about Barb and Brad and the magic they shared. What do you think, Brad?" And Brad said yes, the way he always says yes to adventures, with a twinkle in his eye, and so I got to think about how this Chapter 5 was going to look. And over the course of our annual Yellow Point Lodge holiday, I started talking to the many couples who have held onto each other, and I asked them if they would talk to me about the magic. Most said that it wasn't magic at all, just a lot of damn hard work. But many of them agreed to think about it, and I hope that when we talk again, they can get past the part when it was just a lot of damn hard work and they can share their magic stories, because that's what I want to share with you readers.

I suspect that I will learn a lot from these veterans of committed intimate relationships. I think I might learn, first, what was hard in these long time relationships. Then what wasn't so hard, and then, if I'm lucky, what was cherished. I don't expect to find out the SIX THINGS couples must do to stay together. I think that those six things change with every different match of personalities that come together. But I do think that I will hear some amazing stories, and it just might be true that, as these lovely folks recall the moments of magic and charm, and memories are rekindled, there may be a re awakening of heart flutters and secret looks. I will let you know.

So a year later, I have had the pleasure of spending time with some incredible couples, all of whom have been together 30 plus years. I was a little off on what I thought I would learn, but not too far. These are their stories.

Summer 2011

Anne and Bill had a fairly brief romance before getting married at 19 and 21 years of age. Children followed very soon after, two sons, and Bill began his career in law policing while Ann stayed in touch with her work place two days a week working outside the home on Bill's days off. The boys were very active in sports, lacrosse in particular, and as they got older and better at lacrosse, they were invited to travel around the world for tournaments.

Bill spent 37 years in law enforcement before retiring. The boys grew up in the same family home and the family was active in the community. Going from active parents to empty nesters was easily transitioned for Ann and Bill as they made their home a place for young athletes from around the world to stay while in town at various tournaments. These young adults had met Ann and Bill's sons during their travels. The hosting that Ann and Bill did, they both agreed, was pivotal in keeping them young and involved. They built excellent relationships with these young world traveling athletes, and Ann recalls with a smile on her face, hearing a knock on the door any time of the day or night, and opening it to find a young weary traveler with lacrosse gear stowed away in a backpack, explaining that at least one of their sons had promised a soft bed and a warm meal for as long as was needed.

Ann and Bill continue to have visitors regularly, and they are still so young at heart. Forty eight years later, Ann and Bill still look at each other with a twinkle in their eye. They laugh together, and they clearly enjoy one another's company. The secret to their success as a couple??? Well, they don't really know. No one thing. Lots of things,

and it changes!

Update 2021
Ann and Bill

Ann and Bill continue to live in their family home, although Bill has suffered 2 major strokes and has lost the art of speaking. He and Ann have worked out a way to communicate which sometimes leaves one or the other laughing at the ridiculousness of all of this- Ann and Bill's children and grandchildren are very much a part of their lives and they are still as active as they can be, watching the grandsons' high level lacrosse games as often as they are able.

Summer 2011

Evvie and Bill celebrated their 55th wedding anniversary recently. They met in high school and started falling for each other at the graduation dance in grade 12. Evvie says that she knew right away that she was going to marry Bill, but it still took her 5 years to convince him! Evvie was a teacher and Bill was in law enforcement, later becoming the Chief of Police in his home city.   They were married for 15 years before having their only and beloved child. In the early years, Evvie and Bill didn't see much of each other except on holidays because they worked different shifts, and were often more like two ships passing in the night. Evvie did not pick up teaching again after becoming a mom. Fifty five years later you just don't often see Evvie without Bill. They were not able to tell me or any rituals or practices that they had that kept the fires of romance burning. Evvie simply said, "Divorce was never an option. Murder? Yes, but divorce, no!" The secret to the longevity of their relationship AND the fact that they still want to spend time with each other? Well they didn't really know. No one thing. Lots of things really, and it changes.

Update 2021
Evvie and Bill

Evvie passed away some years ago. Bill lives on his own at 92, with loving support from his son, Liam. They still holiday together and Bill still enjoys a good game of poker with a good scotch to sip on. He can still make me laugh, and he has a huge circle of friends. And of course he misses her.

Summer 2010-

Gord and Marilyn have the longest intact relationship of any of the couples I interviewed, being together for 64 years. Marilyn is one year younger than Gord, and they first met when she sat behind him in grade 1. They have one son who is in his early 60s. Gord had a long and distinguished career and was in the very highest echelons in surveillance work which required them to change their living locations. Upon Gord's retirement they eventually returned to their original home, and still live close to where they met. When I asked the two of them if they had any secrets, they looked at me like I was crazy. Gord said that Marilyn was the nicest and kindest person he had ever known and that she took real good care of him. Marilyn said, with a big smile on her face, "Well, Gord is such a great guy and it was always a lot of fun!" What did they think they did that made their relationship last? Well, they didn't really know. Nothing special! No one thing. Lots of things, and it changes.

Update 2021
Marilyn and Gord

Both Marilyn and Gord have passed on. They were true to each other to the very end. They lived everyday, I think, for each other, and I can still remember Marilyn telling Gord to put a hat on in the sun. Gord was kind of a slow mover by that time, and he would look at those around him as if to say - "Really? A hat? Does she even remember what I did for a living?" Right to the end, they had each other, which is all they seemed to need. I miss them.

Summer 2010

Jim and Edie married in 1950 on a Tuesday evening in October at St. Giles United Church in Vancouver BC. They married on a Tuesday because, they said, the weekend bookings for weddings were booked far in advance, and they didn't want to wait any longer once they had made up their minds! They met at the YMCA in their 20's after Jim first spotted Edie on the bus on her way home from work. Somehow he figured out her name and that they both belonged to the YMCA in Vancouver. He kept trying to book a game of badminton with her as his partner, but apparently Jim was well known for his badminton skills. Edie said that people kept asking if they could take her place as his partner and she kept saying "Sure!", but they seemed destined to be together. Edie had 4 children in 5 years and worked full time in various secretarial positions which was unusual for the time (being a married woman with children), while Jim was a teacher for 35 years. They always worked alongside one another in home-based projects, taking on big tasks such as painting the house or building a carport. The house was always full of kids and pets, and there was always room at the supper table for one more. What kept Jim around for all those years, even in the tough times? "Well" said Jim, "there was really never any question once the kids came along. We were a family" As to the secret to success? No secret, you just keep doing it.

Update 2021 - Edie and Jim

Edie and Jim are my parents, who agree to the interview, very skeptical of this whole idea. Still, they were married nearly sixty years before mom passed. Dad lived another 9 years and in that time he became very very close to me and Kevin, and to the girls. He never considered remarrying, but he was a hopeless romantic and always enjoyed the presence and company of women, when he could get it. Except for the last 3 weeks, he lived on his own, with support, and died so peacefully and beautifully that the memory of it still captures my breath. I miss them both. I am so grateful for the life they gave me, which has led me in so many remarkable directions!

Summer 2010 -

Even though none of the couples could articulate the ingredients necessary to maintaining a long lasting loving and hot love relationship, this is what I think I've learned from them, and seem to me to be the keys to keeping it alive. As well, it may be true that intimate conversations may not have been commonplace between couples of past generations.

1. None of the couples ever even contemplated a divorce. As Evvie said, "Murder yes, divorce, no." They married for life.
2. They enjoyed each other, and still do, after all these years. They still have moments that are private. It might be true that when they look into each other's eyes they feel a sense of peace and calmness. They feel whole.
3. They laughed together.
4. They had good friends that they would regularly get together with and laugh with.
5. They got involved in their kids' lives as much as they could, and had a plan of sorts for when they were going to be empty nesters. They made sure that they still knew each other when the kids were gone.
6. They did family things and things as a family.
7. They had deep, deep feelings of respect for each other.
8. They believed in each other.
9. Each felt a sense of honor being the other one's partner.
10. They seemed to know who was in charge of what. Another way to say that is that each of the partners was territorial. For the most part, men were the main providers financially, but the women were respected and even revered for their domains within the home and the marriage. Both parties

had their unique skills and their abilities. The men did not step where the women reigned, and vice versa (until retirement) .

11. They made good family memories. Even when things were tough, they made sure that they had fun times together.
12. They somehow found time for each other. This was not consistent, nor did any of them say that this was at the top of their lists, but the time they did find to spend with each other away from the madness of daily life or kids or whatever was good.
13. Sometimes they went to bed still mad at each other.
14. Both of them believe in a future together.
15. Each expected to take care of their partner. Edie would say, "Each partner has to give better than 50/50. It has to be at least 60/60."

And perhaps the last questions we should be reflecting on when things become challenging in a relationship, as they do for all of us is, "Who do I want to grow old with?" "How long do I want to be mad?" "How much of my energy do I want to spend on this?" Being angry with someone you care deeply about is exhausting, and can have dire health and wellness consequences over the long haul. We can pretty easily get stuck on something, some act or some phraseology that cuts us deep to the heart and can lead to "cognitive distortion" or thinking gone wrong.

Psychologists use the term "cognitive distortions" to describe irrational, inflated thoughts or beliefs that distort a person's perception of reality, usually in a negative way. Cognitive distortions are common but can be hard to recognize if you don't know what to look for. Many occur as automatic thoughts. They are so <u>habitual</u> that the thinker often doesn't realize he or she has the power to change them. Many grow to believe that's just the way things are. (Good Therapy: Cognitive Distortions. John Tagg 1996)

This "thinking gone wrong" where one gets stuck in a thinking feedback loop which is unhealthy and leaves little to no opportunity to break out of can be adjusted but requires working with a person trained in Cognitive Behavioral Therapy. The most important thing to remember is that the time invested in healing is worth its weight in gold. A life partner is a gift that needs tending to and happy attention.

Long term relationships take an investment by both partners in every way. No one gets there without spending considerable time. Good relationships are healthy relationships, where each party not only gets something out of it, but is better because of it. Good relationships evolve and grow and change. Needs change, challenges change. What was hard when the children were young is very different from what's hard when the children are teens. Health issues become more prevalent as we age, and before we start worrying about whether we are going to have to take care of this person next to us as he or she ages, we better be prepared to face the fact that it is just as likely that it will be you who is the one needing to be cared for. For these lovely folks, "I DO" meant, "I buy the whole package, the warts and the wonderful. I buy it all". One person said to me, when a man marries a woman, he thinks that the woman who stands before him at the altar will always look like that. When a woman marries a man, she thinks that she can change the little things that drive her crazy about him, over time. Well, surprise surprise, they are both wrong! We may look different over time, but the package pretty much remains the same. It had better feel pretty good for both parties to start with.

Cindy and Kevin - over 4 decades together
So it's my turn now to talk about us. You already know a lot, including the timeline the writing of this book has spanned. As I try to figure out what happened to my interest and determination to carry on with this project, I realize that, once I was rejected from about 9 different publishers and could not find a project supporter in that crowd, I lost faith in my idea. The bottom kind of dropped out of my energy around it. I doubted myself. I let other things come along and capture my interest, and I only thought about this book when someone asked me about it. I would sort of look at my shoes and say something like, Ya, it's on the back burner right now, I'm busy with ….."

That lack of interest in carrying on with the project did not, however, stop the inquiries and the fun to be had around talking about six Minute Sex. I made up (or copied?) a saying, a reminder really, about something I called Frisky Friday! Frisky Friday was meant as a gentle reminder to us long term people that it was that time of week again- think about it!!! At work I would often say to staff in the Friday bulletin or in the Friday afternoon closing circle, "Don't forget -it's FRISKY FRIDAY!!!!" It became a bit of a game for a long time, and then I was challenged by a coworker one day. She said, "Cindy, is it ALWAYS Frisky Friday for you guys on Fridays or what? And with a smile on my face, I said something like, "Of course not, but at our age it counts if we even think about it!" More laughter. So then the saying switched to, "OK, it's Frisky Friday, and remember if you're my age it counts even if you think about it!!" More ways to have fun, more ways to remember that you can take some time for intimacy, anytime, really.

So, I recently retired - well, to be truthful, I retired on December 31 2020, in the midst of COVID, when it was clear that my health had taken all the hits it could. I missed so much work and was unable to work full time, and it became clear that it was time to take care of me. As well, the position I held really required that I be present on the job, at work everyday, and I just was not well enough to attend full time. So, with a heavy heart, I contacted HR and made arrangements to finish my career earlier than I had planned. But, in the end, it was totally the RIGHT decision as I have been a picture of wellness since my days have become my own. My retirement date meant that I could ski full time all that winter, where the Frisky Fridays continued (and in fact got BETTER) and kept us laughing and thinking about it!! As well, "Frisky Friday" may become a folk legend as the phrase made it into the retirement farewell event hosted by the school district recently (2022), and everyone was at first curious, and then had a good laugh! I am so grateful for the career I had, and will remember the kids and the staffs and the families with love in my heart forever!

And for us? What keeps us together? Well, like everyone else, lots of things and no one thing. Except to say that I am not really sure why Kevin fell in love with me in the first place. On the outside, he was so cute (still is), he was sexy, he had a motorcycle, he loved camping, he knew his music, he could spit (this is an art form, one that I have never learned), he knew lots of guys and was a "guy's guy", he held a good steady job with good pay and benefits, he put down the toilet seat without being reminded, he loved cats (and dogs we found out later), he had lots of friends and was a real catch. And on the inside, he was sensitive, a patient and attentive lover, he was ok with my early wildness and forgave me when I made mistakes. He waited for me to complete my career training and charmed my parents and the rest of my family and friends with his natural ability to be interesting and attentive. Like most couples I think, we struggled through the times when intimacy and physical closeness was something we thought about as we fell asleep, but all through it we tried to stay closely connected with date nights and special celebrations. When the kids were babies we hired a babysitter and the two of us went to the living room, just to spend some time together. And here we are, with a healthy dose of romance still lingering in our loins.

Not so long ago we went on a cruise for a week - our first cruise ever. It was awesome. I remember saying after we got home, "Hey Kev, I didn't know that there could be 4 Frisky Fridays in one week!!!!" But, last week we got a puppy - so as for Frisky Fridays? It counts if you just think about it!!!

So, a couple of lessons I have learned:

1. Rejection. My manuscript was rejected by about 9 different publishers, and I let that end my efforts. It makes me think about how many times I have rejected the loving advances that Kevin has made over the years, and the effect that has had to have had on our intimate relationship. Let me tell you, it was way more than 9 times - something to think about as we age together. Thank God he never gave up on me.

2. Don't let anyone or anything take the wind out of your sails when you have an idea that makes you smile. Keep at it, or at least go back to it.

3. Feel really good about your long term relationship. Feel proud and warm and loving - this commitment stuff is hard at times.

Chapter Six

SOME MORE IDEAS, AND FUN CONSIDERATIONS IN SUPPORT OF SIX MINUTE SEX

During the journey of writing this book, we have had many, many laughs about the number and variety of offshoots this book seems to present as opportunities! One rainy November afternoon many years ago, I remember saying to my husband that he was likely going to be the envy of many men. After all, what wife and partner of 28 years writes a book promoting Six Minute Sex??

He then suggested that he write a sequel called, "The Real Truth about Six Minute Sex" where he dispels the myth that he and I take advantage of every six minute time slot that comes up. In fact, we still sometimes revert back to the desert and oasis model.

My sequel would then be, "Why Women Don't Want Sex Right After the Family Dog Dies" or "Don't Try to Comfort me with

Sex: The Dog Just Died" or "Proof that Men Really are From Mars and Women Really Are From Venus: How Each Gender Handles the Death of the Family Dog".

His sequel to that sounds something like, "There's Always Going to Be a Reason to Say No to Six Minutes", and my return sequel is something like "Six Minutes to Separation". Sound familiar??

The truth is, for many couples, we need to consciously make the time for intimacy with each other, and yes things do come up (like the family dog / cat/ lizard/ bird/ horse /etc. dies, health issues, changes in family, other sadnesses, crises and losses, guests that come and stay and stay and stay…) that just throws a wet towel onto everything and makes anything more than just existing feel like too much work. However, getting close sooner rather than later will leave all of us feeling better about pretty much everything. Retreating inward, while necessary for most of us, is not where we should stay for too long. It is lonely and dark and cold.

Sadness and intimacy actually do go together as we try to make sense of losses and share our feelings, some of which have no words. That closeness allows us to let our guards down and empty out some of the sadness that seems overwhelming. It is not a betrayal to feel good and close and intimate in times of sadness. If you can manage it, try it. You might surprise yourself.

So in response to my husband's idea of intimacy so soon after our beloved dog died, I should have said yes. I should have said yes, right here, right now, the sooner the better. Clothes on or off. Because I would have felt better, not good, but better. And for my husband, who like many men has trouble expressing just how deeply he was saddened by the loss of something or someone he loves, I know it would have helped him, he would have felt better, and our intimacy and understanding of one another would have deepened. Yes, he would have felt better in a different way than I would have, but I may have perhaps helped him heal a little bit faster, and we would have shared something special, where he got to lead the sadness. I will know for next time.

Sometimes Things Just don't Work Out!

Have you ever heard people in relationship say: "Well, we never go to bed mad at each other!"

Really??

Well, I have. We have. And I always feel myself shrink a little when I hear someone make such an incredible declaration! I am in awe! So is Kevin. Because we have gone to bed, mad at each other, many times over the 40 plus years we have been together. Many times. We've even woken up still mad! We've slept apart, not just on the couch or in the guest room, but in different abodes when we've been really cheezed off with the other. And to be fair, it is me who is usually creating the drama, often because of feeling, for a long time, unheard or ignored or misunderstood. Or just lonely for some love.

I remember when Kevin was changing careers and enrolled in a very challenging technical program. He was so focussed on his program he forgot about me. One Friday evening, without really telling him, I planned a very special date night, complete with all the trimmings. When he arrived home I had the music tuned in to our favorites, the pots cooking and tempting smells coming out of the oven. I think he tried to focus on us and being loving. I really do. But he had some electrical engineering problem to solve and, right after we finished eating, he called our neighbor who was an electrical /electronic engineer and asked if he could go over to discuss it with him. So - he left. Dishes still on the table! So much for date and romance night! I was so hurt and so mad, I grabbed the dog and the dog food, and went to my parents house. Left a note saying not to look for me.

Remember that ANGER is a strength - based emotion. We use the emotion of anger to protect our soft, vulnerable underbelly of emotions such as embarrassment, hurt, and vulnerability to name a few. Always try to check in with yourself what emotion you are feeling, and behavior you are displaying to convey that emotion.

I arrived at mom and dad's in tears. I made them promise to say that I wasn't there should he call, even though they felt pretty uncomfortable about being dishonest. I spent the weekend feeling sorry for myself, building many sandcastle plans in my head about what my future would now look like. I was pampered and spoiled by my mom, who seemed to understand my disappointment. My dad stayed pretty quiet.

Sunday came, as did the phone call I knew would come. This was long before call display, and of course my mom answered it. I could tell from the look on her face who she was talking to. She put her hand over the mouthpiece and looked at me with pleading eyes and said, "He knows you're here. He drove by." I walked out of the room and said over my shoulder, 'I'll leave the room - then you won't be lying!'

I had fully supported this change in his career- in fact I was the head cheerleader - but I didn't plan on being ignored and left out. I thought, as I often did, that Kevin should be able to handle everything - all responsibilities! And that was not fair, I later learned. We all have our threshold, and those thresholds vary.

It's hard to stay mad. At least I find it hard, especially when there was no intention for Kevin to be hurtful. Feeling hurt is much easier. I wonder why? I know that, when Kevin takes on a project, it often requires a big time commitment on a tight timeline, so his focus is like a spotlight. And this was a big project that was added to an already full agenda. He was changing his career half way through his career years. He had old school training - he was supposed to be the provider. I was a contributor, but he was the provider! So, he took his coursework seriously in order to be successful in his new venture. And it was my judgment that the upgrade was interfering with my needs.

Anyway, the story had a happy ending. I stayed two more nights at my mom and dad's. I decided 2 more nights were a good compromise - he could work uninterrupted on his courses and coursework and I could kind of (figuratively) fall back into the loving and patient arms of my parents! I had my lunch made for me, complete with the extra special treats of chopped veggies and 2 cookies wrapped in wax paper! I slept in my old bed and my coffee was made in the morning. I had to go out to buy some new clothes to wear to work, which we could ill afford, but I kept it to the minimum, knowing I was going home soon.

So we talked. I was able to articulate my feelings and the reasons for feeling hurt, and while Kevin would not commit to being able to change his focus before he finished his courses, he did remind me that this change was my idea, and asked me if I wanted him to quit so he could spend more time with me. It sounded so stupid when he said it that way - so childish, that I laughed out loud. He did intentionally outline his course commitments to me, giving me an overview of timelines and expectations. We carved out a bit of space for togetherness, and I stopped expecting him to be available for me, at least on that particular time frame.

So, we are not on the "Never go to bed mad at each other" list. Nor are we on the "and we never fight, argue or disagree" list! However, we have made a deal that we each get to decide how long we are going to stay mad at the other one about something, and this change has been a huge hit! Anger with bookends (or hurt, or embarrassment, or upset that comes across as anger with bookends)! It's great! We get to be as mad as we want for as long as we choose! The rules state that you have to let the partner know how long you intend on staying mad for. You can shorten the timeline, but you cannot lengthen it without discussion. Of course, at the start partners tend to set ridiculous timelines. "I'm going to be mad at you for 2 weeks!" But that is a long time to stay mad, because anger takes a lot of energy and comes with particular kinds of behaviors that are difficult to maintain! The silent treatment is the easiest I find, but as the emotion gets old, I find myself wanting to tell Kevin a story about something that has happened, or pass on a hello from a mutual friend. It's much easier to stay mad at someone you don't live your life with, so anywhere from 10 minutes to 4 hours seems to be our norm.

It is such a marvelous strategy that I incorporated this skill into my whole life! Mad at a friend for missing a date, mad at a coworker for not siding with you, a boss for making a change you disagree with - the only rule is that you have to let the other know you are mad (just in case there was a misunderstanding on yours or their part), and then you have to decide how long you are going to spend energy being mad, or hurt or upset - whatever label you use. It's smart, it's healthy - it's anger with bookends!

Emotional Bank Account

Dr. Scott Stanley (Psychology Today Dec 2019) brings up some really great considerations that challenge us in our relationship with our true love. These are challenges that we have some control over, but can sometimes get the best of us because, let's face it, we all have a lot of control over an action or a reaction. For example, forgiveness is something we choose to do, or not to do in relationship. Forgiveness requires us to overlook something that has happened, that impacts negatively on our feelings for the other. Sometimes forgiveness is easy - for example I forgive you for putting my red jumper into the wash with the white laundry (even though everything has turned pink); I forgive you for forgetting to check the oil level in the car (even though you could have seized the engine); I forgive you for working late on this important date (even though we had plans) or I forgive you for promising to pick up the drycleaning and then forgetting (even though I was counting on wearing that suit tomorrow). Sometimes forgiveness is hard or even in some cases seems impossible. For many, there are some acts that seem unforgivable. Everyone knows their own personal boundaries for forgiving because forgiveness is a choice. It does not mean forgetting, it means overlooking and moving forward. Often it means adjusting plans in the future to avoid repeating the same behaviors. So as a reminder to myself, and to build up my "Emotional Bank Account" with my chosen partner, I need to remember that it's the little things that count - the little acts of kindness and compassion, of trust and love. And these "deposits" that I make into his Emotional Bank Account (and he to mine) do not have to be tangible or hands on. For example, I try to make a point of listening more to better understand where he stands on certain issues, what kinds of things never slip his mind, and what things will never ever stick in his memory because it just doesn't register on his "matter meter". I can figure out, for myself, what behaviors I can let go, and what behaviors are a hard no. I can stop testing him and trust that he loves me as much as I love him. And I can communicate with him my list of things that are "hard no's". I can support him with things he is trying or working at, I can ask about progress or challenges - I can invest in his interests, AND I can communicate mine. Remember that, all those little deposits in the Emotional Bank Account grow and become big. They earn interest! They form the foundation that allows us to become more able to sustain things that inevitably come along in life that require the two of us to face the challenge together, such as the loss of loved ones, forced retirement or relocation, financial crisis and other potential hardships. They become the rock upon which we can stand together. Things we need to work for in long term relationships - it's worth it!

Commitment to your partner - You can show your commitment by some tangible act like inviting your partner to do something with you that you both enjoy. You can look for ways to provide more emotional or tangible support to your partner around an ongoing personal struggle.

Honesty - There is no greater act of respect than being honest with your partner - with your heart and your head. That doesn't mean you need to hurt your partner's feelings when you are honest about something that might be delicate. Feedback that can be hurtful is always softer when the intention is to support and make things better - but at the same time you must own your own stuff. By that I mean you must have the courage to be fallible and imperfect and own your behavior when it has not been so noble. We do this as a couple by listening carefully to our partner, taking time to understand the intention behind the feedback, taking responsibility for mistakes we have made, and then vowing to do better (and then of course doing better). But this is a two way street! If we start by celebrating the things that we LOVE about each other, the hard stuff becomes less hard. Making a deposit or many deposits in the Emotional Bank Account first better sustains the foundation of the relationship during tougher times.

Forgiveness (as mentioned above) is so important. I once was told - the act of forgiving gives us a lightness in our hearts that cannot be matched - and forgive does not mean forget - it means "I/we can move on".

And the other side of Forgiveness

Accepting kindness and generosity - Why is it so much easier to give than to receive? If a person has found the grace in their heart to forgive you for something you did, then the rudest thing you can do is refuse the forgiveness offered. (Tibetan Saying).

Empathy - being kind, gentle and understanding, even when it's hard, is an elixir for your partner. They may need your strength and understanding from time to time, rather than your judgment.

Listening without distraction - You can decide to listen more to your partner. You can work at articulating more clearly what you want.

Show and express your joy of being together - You can show joy about something your partner has achieved. You can show and express delight when you or your partner finish something you have been working on, start something new and exciting or surprise each other with something new!

It's the little things that matter - pay attention to them. They then naturally mature and turn into good big things.

Shame: A Most Challenging Emotion

Over my career, I have been fortunate enough to have my attention captured by the emotion and the judgment of shame - a tremendously complex feeling. Shame, as a noun, is defined in the Oxford Languages Dictionary as "a partial feeling of humiliation caused by the consciousness of wrong or foolish behavior". Associated words include humiliation, mortification, embarrassment, and guilt. It means you feel regretful about something you have done or caused.

As a verb, the Oxford Languages definition reads: (of a) person, action or situation, to make someone feel ashamed. Associated words include humiliate, mortify, embarrass, put someone in their place. This means that shame is used to judge another person's actions.

The fundamental difference between the verb and the noun is this - As a noun, shame is something that someone does to themselves when they feel they have done something very wrong - they feel like a bad person. As a verb, shaming is something that someone does to another person - shames that person for some action. The emotion of shame produces autonomic responses: the head drops as the back neck muscles lose strength, eyes close and the body curves in on itself as if trying to be invisible. As well, shame can produce the flight, fight or freeze response, which is protective. Why does this matter in the context of this book? Well, a person feeling shame about an action they committed is bad enough - that is when you beat yourself up about something you have done and feel like a bad person. However, being shamed by someone you love is humiliating and debilitating, and it ruins relationships. Shame shuts things down. If someone is trying to shame you, call them on it. If you are feeling shame or ashamed of something you have done, own it and ask for forgiveness. Do that with intention. That is a healthy path out of shame.

On a lighter note....

What can we do to maintain the intimacy in our long term relationship?

"G" rated ideas to stay close

In keeping with the whimsical theme of this book, and understanding the importance of intimacy balanced with fun, and making time in our busy lives, there needs to be a whole host of other fun things we can do with our partners on the spur of the moment that support, lead to or enhance intimacy with our life partners. And not all of them need to be done behind closed doors.

There are six levels of these kinds of activities. These are:

1. Momentary, short lived, "G" rated
2. Momentary, short lived "R" rated
3. Short term, semi sustained public behavior
4. Active action-packed activity
5. Surprise opportunities
6. Long sweet kisses, or long sexy kisses

Some examples of each of these levels included:

Momentary, short lived "G" rated touches - try them out!

1. Gentle hand touches such as on the shoulder, under the forearm, on the cheek, at the waist
2. Arms on the shoulders
3. Leaning on the other, gently
4. Nose to nose with a kind word
5. Hugs
6. The long lean in

When the kids were younger, one day in the chaos of the morning, I dashed out very, very early with one of my daughters, trying to fit in a 7:00a.m. grocery shop before work and school. As it happened, my husband stopped into the same store and went through the same cash register we did, shortly after us. He called out to me as we were on our way to the exit, and I was delighted to see him when I turned around. In our banter, I said, "Hey, I know you! Didn't I sleep with you last night?" and we both had a laugh. And as much as this may have shocked the cashier, she too smiled, and we carried on our day. It was just a moment, in fact it was a "G" rated intimate moment where we celebrated our connection.

Momentary short lived "R" rated actions. RISKY!! These behaviors are fun and can be done privately in public, when no one's looking. If you choose to engage in this way, be prepared to be caught and live with the embarrassment!

1. Gentle bum pinch, pat or squeeze
2. Flashing
3. Shimmy hugs
4. Little lap dance
5. A tweak
6. Risky rude gesture

Short term, semi sustained public behavior
1. Arm link
2. Hand holding
3. Arms around each other

4. Human footrest on the couch in front of the TV or while reading
5. Foot massage
6. Head on shoulder

Active, action-packed activity

1. Close dancing to a favorite song on the radio, in the kitchen, or the RV, the boat, or ?? for a few moments
2. Racing each other to somewhere close like to the car, to the kitchen, to the table, and trying to hold the other back from winning. This needs to be done gently.
3. Tag
4. Wrestling
5. Keep away
6. Chair dancing - in your own chair

Surprise opportunities

1. Seeing each other out in public by surprise, act as delighted to see each other as you would be an old and dear friend. Smile, hug, kiss, hold hands for a moment, go on your way!
2. Say thank you and provide a peck on the cheek for jobs the other does as a regular household job or responsibility. Do it by surprise!
3. On a check in phone call, say "I'm so happy you phoned. I was hoping you might have six minutes for me a little later``. Put a smile on your face when you say it. A smile travels through the phone.

4. "Stop and look at me when I say this". Then stop dead, grab the other one by the shoulders and say something memorable like, "Wow, you still have the most gorgeous eyes in the world!".
5. I'm not busy, you're not busy - let's sit with a coffee and visit! Be sure you take the time BEFORE you get busy!
6. Remind your partner of a time you had together that was super special. Say,"Hey honey! Remember when we…" you will both feel the warmth of the lovely memory and may even plan something similar!

During our first trip to Mexico in 1983, we had the unfortunate experience of being robbed on our first day. One of the big items taken was our Travelers Cheques. Of course we had the kind that had replacement insurance, but we had a great deal of difficulty finding a way to report the theft and get the Traveler's Cheques replaced. Remember, this was in the early '80's, when the World Wide Web was yet to become a reality. After several attempts, we were told by some guy in a bank that we could probably get replacement cheques at the big airport, as we were traveling through Mexico city airport on our way from Vera Cruz to the west coast. So, with my pigeon Spanish (which was marginally better than Kevin's), I joined the line at the first bank/cambio exchange center in the Mexico city airport we came to. There were several. In Spanish, Traveler's Cheques translates as Cheques Viajeros, which is the phrase I used with the tellers. Every time I got to the front of a line and said "Cheques Viajeros?", she or he would point me to the next line up at the next bank, so I would get in the next lineup and pose the same question once I reached the teller. I finally ran out of patience having received the same instruction over and over, so I babysat the luggage while Kevin took over the lining up. After a couple of hours with the same results, we gave up. We decided that, at least we had recovered the peso equivalent that we had lost, and while we were not comfortable carrying around that much cash, clearly we were not going to find Traveler's Cheques. Much later we discovered that Kevin had been asking for Cheques Huevos or "Egg Cheques", and had gotten the exact same results as I had asking for Travelers Cheques!! It still makes us laugh today, thinking of Kevin asking for egg cheques and being sent to the next line up!!!

7. Call one another an endearing name, out of the blue! The other day Kevin called me his sunshine. Later in the day I sent him a message reminding him that he did that. I got back a burst of hearts!!

8. Finding an old romantic photo of the two of you that has great memories, and recall and retell the story behind the photo to each other

Long sweet kisses, long sexy kisses
There is perhaps nothing more surprising or flattering than when your long term partner surprises you with a long sweet kiss when traditionally, kissing in your relationship meant a peck on the lips or cheek, or just a quick acknowledgement. Try it! Suddenly, the kiss shifts from sweet to sexy. The one being surprised thinks, "Oh! Well! HMMM! Maybe?". Both of

you are thinking of other possibilities. Even though nothing may come of it, it is the thought that is fun and exciting!

And don't be afraid to be public about how you feel about one another. Getting closer does mean touching each other. Yes, touching. Public touching should not embarrass anyone, or make anyone who witnesses such acts feel as if they are interfering in something private. Touch, in the right way, with the right intention, can be so sensuous, reassuring, and supportive. Many people love to be touched in loving ways. This is different from being groped, or being fully engaged in some foreplay touching. So for example, you likely should not be groping your partner on a park bench - that gives most of us the "yuk" feeling when we see it in others, prompting response like "Get a room!". This touching game is so easy and takes only reminding yourself to do it differently. And it's ok to copy. When you see another couple playing the touching game, it can spark your ideas and you can copy them. You might wonder if they too have read the Six Minute Sex Book (they probably have!), and see that it's really working for them! However don't dismiss the park bench yet. A head on a shoulder, holding hands, reading a book or an article to the other - this is what only 2 people can do. While others might think it looks a little silly, your behavior might give them some ideas for themselves. Neither partner is allowed to expect any of these spontaneous actions to be done everyday, or every week, or every anything. These are not meant to be expectations, but rather little lovelies, surprises that make us feel closer and desire to be more intimate.

Gentle touching also lets our partner see our vulnerability. A hand on the chest, the cheek or the back is warming and reassuring, and depicts intimacy even in the largest of crowds. And when others of us see that kind of touching going on between long term partners, it makes us feel good, and perhaps a little envious. When I see a couple (to be fair, usually an older couple, or a couple with a couple of kids in tow) holding hands as they walk in public, I always think wonderful things. And when my husband grabs my hand in public, I feel loved and proud and flattered. Who knew that such a little thing could make such a difference!

Date Night: Should have led with this advice!!

These rendezvous are much more important than we ever thought. You don't really even have to go anywhere! Date nights help us remember those old "hot steamy" date nights that we had at the beginning, and provide the fuel to replicate, on some small scale, those feelings! Like early days sex and old people's sex, date nights in long term relationships look different from early relationship date nights. There are some very important rules to follow to be sure that we all make the most of those special times.

Rules

So, let's say that you and your partner have planned a special evening together, a date night! Date night should include some time for intimacy. It always used to, so why not? Some couples are able to maintain a date night once a week or once a month, where they parcel off a chunk of time to spend with each other. Eating, drinking and visiting are fine and you can do most of those things on the run, even with the kids around, however Date Night should include some kind of six minute interlude, not by chance but by design. So the advice provided which should become a rule is this: **have sex first, before anything else.** I'm not kidding - Have sex **FIRST!**

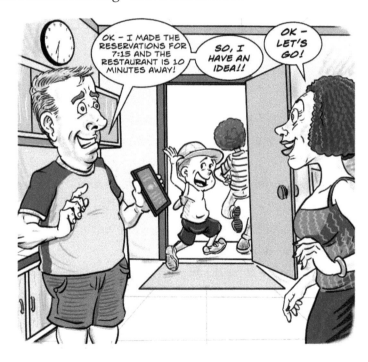

Everyone agrees with this rule, but doesn't always follow it, and guess what! The lovely evening ends without having consummated the date! No one starts out the date thinking

Cindi Seddon

that this is a no sex date. In fact, some couples have cute, kinky, tantalizing ideas that include naughty underwear, catch phrases or other messages passed between them that are intended to heighten the sense of urgency and excitement over the course of the evening. However, when couples wait until later, more often than not, the next day dawns without anyone having any sexual satisfaction. Here are the excuses I've heard.

1. Timing

Life just has a way of jumping up and getting in our way. Even the best of plans can get postponed and canceled. Kids need to be picked up after the date, someone calls, a last minute memory of uncompleted work taps us on the shoulder and so on. Starting with six minutes ensures that this part is taken care of.

2. Ate, drank too much and now I'm too sleepy

That great bottle of wine together with the martini before dinner, coupled with a full belly of great food is almost a guarantee of the sleeping disease hitting harder than the hot, hot six minutes you've been talking about all night. Let's face it, in the first 18 months of a relationship, nothing would stop the two of you from finishing everyday with a romp in the hay. Now, however, the bath just isn't that hot anymore!

3. Shut Up! Just Shut Up!

I have a friend who tried to practise the "have sex first" rule, because she says, every time they leave it for later, her and her hubby will get onto some contentious topic during the date, she will get angry or frustrated, and her thoughts go from HOT to NOT on your life are we having sex tonight. "Just Shut Up. Stop Talking. This is going Nowhere Good!" she thinks, as the conversation heats up, not as in foreplay but as in disagreement. Having sex first releases all of those lovely endorphins, and chances are those controversial topics won't even come up!

4. The Intimacy sets tone for the date

Too much preparation is no good either. When date night starts with an hour of kitchen prep, food prep, and other detailed minutia, momentum can be lost. DON'T fall into that trap. That is "good intentions gone wrong". Find each other first. Order pizza for the kids BEFORE you get home. Tell them that it is date night. Set those Rules of Interruption early, then follow them. Plan the food and the drinks so it doesn't take an hour to set this thing up. Meet and hold each other first. Get lost in each other's eyes. It makes all the difference when you prepare for intimacy, not for eating or drinking or anything else.

PLAN FOR EVERYTHING ELSE SECOND. HAVE SEX FIRST! HAVE FAITH THAT IT WILL WORK OUT WELL.

Having sex first is just a good idea. You want to be closer to your partner afterward. Have you ever noticed a couple out for the evening who just can't seem to get enough of each other?   And you think, "Wow, they're in for a good time tonight?" Well, here's the secret. They have ALREADY HAD sex, and there just may be more in store for them for later on. These folks have figured out the secret and they are not telling anyone. Well, now you know. Having sex first makes EVERYTHING better, including appetite, and there may even be another round in store for the both of you.

A final couple of stories where lessons were learned that made a difference to us, you might relate!

Renovations –

Oh Boy! What a Pandora's Box! It all seems like a good idea at the time! Lovingly, as a partnership, you plan out an exciting renovation that will transform some part or parts of your living space.   You determine how cooking, dishes, laundry will get done. You pack up things that you don't think you are going to need and happily welcome the start date. And trust me when I say it will all end up great - it's just the "getting to great" that will suck every ounce of patience, love, understanding and the ability to picture and dream of the finished project that gets you down a bit. Or, you may have renovations thrust upon you with a kitchen fire or a burst hose in the night (that's what happened to us one time) which, at first, you choose to accept as a bit of a gift of a reno. But 5 months later, plan to be sick of doing dishes in the bathroom sink or cooking on the BBQ's single burner! But all these things - the boat, the RV, the renovations - all of them give us a chance to learn a bit more of each other and to grow together. An unexpected foot rub at the end of a long hard day does wonders to restoring vitality, and possibly opening the door for some quick romance!! Hang on to each other. You started this together, and in the thick of change, there has to be a way through to the other side!

Ends with the story of a Dog: The Jasper Story

Kevin was a pretty easy going guy about pretty much everything, however he had a couple of hard "NO"s. His world, which included never getting married AND never having children, didn't bother me at all. What did I care? Ten months prior I had left an unsuccessful marriage in New Zealand (no kids, no property, just a broken heart) and I had no desire to rush into such a big commitment. So it didn't matter to me. Instead, when I thought of the longevity of this relationship, I knew that, even if it didn;t work out, there were indeed really lovely men in the world, and Kevin was one of them.

Kevin was a tradesman, having followed his father's footsteps into the sheetmetal trade. He had a steady job, he made good money, and was settled. I on the other hand was a full time student, working part time as a grocery cashier and financing my school and life through part time wages and student loans.

He quickly introduced me to his parents, his family and his friends. I did the same with him. We went camping and 4 wheel driving in the bush, and we hiked the mountains and camped some more, and we skied a bit. I loved his hobbies and he loved mine. We did some short trips with me on the back of his motorbike, Completely Thrilling!! He owned a landcruiser, which I thought was the coolest truck in the world, and we had some very exciting and wonderful adventures. Although Kevin never wanted to make long term plans, we did manage to plan a trip to Mexico the second year we were together, and if we needed something to test our relationship, that was the trip to do it!

Being adventurers, we had planned our trip well off the more touristy "beaten path" which proved a problem at many levels. On our first day in Mexico we were robbed!! The thieves came into our room in the afternoon while we slept off our jet lag (and the 2 margaritas). They stole all of our traveler's cheques, our plane tickets and our visitor's visas, which we needed to get out of the country. We ran into roadblock after roadblock trying to get our traveler's cheques replaced, our tickets replaced and our visitors' visas replaced. The story goes on and on, but suffice it to say it was an unbelievable experience. From being chased down the street by the police in Vera Cruz to discovering a secret peek-a boo-hole in the mirror in our beautiful (but remarkably cheap) hotel room (which had a great view of both beds from a linen closet), to missing our flight home, to figuring out that the feds seemed to be trying to set us up for a cocaine bust, it was remarkable. In fact, when we went through customs in Los Angeles, we were followed by undercover officers and thoroughly searched by the border patrol. That trip could have been the end, but in fact it was the beginning. We thought if we could survive that and still laugh about it as we retold the stories, then we were in pretty good shape, and we made a pretty good team. So for the first 11 years Kevin and I were in a committed relationship which morphed into a common law relationship. We certainly had our bumpy times. I finished my degree and finally became a teacher. We bought a house, converted the downstairs into a small suite and rented out our upstairs, which paid a large portion of the mortgage. We were both pet lovers, we had cats, but I well remember the rocky road we had to travel when I said I wanted a dog! I had grown up in a family with a long living dog, and I still dreamed of her regularly.

One day my sister phoned me from the downtown core and told me that,as she was eating her lunch outside her office building that day, she had seen a Golden Retriever running around in traffic who was finally rescued by the SPCA My sister knew I had been wanting a dog, so she suggested I give the Dog Pound a call and see what fate awaited.

Kevin had a completely different idea.

He said he had a dog when he was a kid, maybe even more than one, but no one in the family ever took ownership. And unfortunately, he had no strong and/or happy memories of owning a family dog, just memories of loss and confusion and sadness.

So, Kevin did not want a dog.

I called the Pound and was told that the owner had been in touch and was going to pick his dog up in a couple of days. I thanked them for their information and was about to hang up when the fellow said, "Wait! Often the owners never show up, so if we have a no show, this dog is available for adoption in a week, and you are the first to inquire so you will have first chance! So I had one week, maybe, to sway Kevin into my way of thinking. It was a long week, but the next Saturday we were pulling out of our driveway to go and have a look at the dog. Kevin made one final but flimsy attempt to squash the plans when he expressed concerns that the dog, if we got it, might chew apart and otherwise damage the inside of his newly refurbished truck. It was only by promising that the dog had to feel like a good fit for both of us to bring him home that we carried on.

Jasper was beautiful! He was indeed a golden retriever, about 2 years old, and he was gentle and kind and so appreciative of love and attention. He came home with us that day, and we had him until he was 17. But man, could he be naughty! He was an escape artist and would climb the brand new 6 foot fence, built to keep him in the yard, like it was a low hedge. He would always come home, except if the doggy police found him first. Then, we had to go and pay a hefty fine to bring him home, which we always did. I remember Kevin going to get him one day, and he related this story: (Kevin speaking) When I got to the parking lot and got out of the car, there was a long row of cages, full of other run away dogs, and of course, there was Jasper, looking at me and wagging his tail. I yelled out, "Jasper, you bad dog. You SIT!" so ALL the dogs sat down!"

Jasper had another bad habit of ripping down any curtains when left alone. After he did it a second time, we took down all the curtains, and we never hung them again.

But Jasper was a really great dog. We called him Jabu-Dabi, we called him Jasper the Great Indian Golden Retriever, and made up stories of his adventures, and on other occasions, we called him unprintable names when he was naughty.

Jasper was fiercely loyal. When we would go swimming in the ocean or a lake, he always stuck by my side. Swimming for him was as easy as walking. He would pull me around the lake or ocean - I would just

Cindi Seddon

gently hang onto his tail. I had to abandon learning how to wind surf as Jasper got very worried about me out there on this raft thing, and he would not stop circling the board. I was so worried I was going to drop the kite on his head I just quit. Jasper would jump off the end of a wharf with us and swim around, he would dive down, head fully underwater, to retrieve a stick or a weighted ball - he was our constant companion. We called him Nanny Jasper. When we had babies, we would prop them up on his warm belly and he wouldn't move. As they grew up a bit and became more independent and curious, they would pull his tail, or try to poke him in the eye. He never responded with anything but patience and love. He was a remarkable companion. He was my running partner, my comforter and my friend. I still miss him, and we still tell Jasper stories.

Jasper was the best dog because he taught Kevin and I what unconditional love looked like. He taught us patience, and helped us see the delight in the smallest of things. He showed us what it was to love something else more than your own self. Now, for the first time in many years we are dog-less*, having had to say goodbye to our wonderful GoldenDoodle Goldilocks, just over a year ago - a story I will save for later. Not really sure if another dog is in our future - sad face…

*update - puppy in the house warning - check out SizzlenotFizzle.com for great puppy pictures of our Lovely!

145

The next chapter or addition to this book is in the making as I write. I really want to thank all our readers and listeners for engaging with us in some way or other, and we hope that this kind of whimsical idea has brought a closeness back into your relationship that may have diminished somewhat over time.

Please remember to check and contribute your opinions and ideas to

SIZZLENOTFIZZLE.COM, launching February 14, 2023
 check the site frequently for our top six choices and features in
Sexy songs
Great wine
Delicious craft beer
Great and delicious non alcohol choices and ideas
Great and not so great dating ideas! We'll give you our review!
...and more ideas about Six Minute Sex. Welcome to the club!!!!